KISS Guide to Crystal Healing

(Keep It Simple Spirit)

Diane Bloom

Dedication

Books are never written in a vacuum and they are certainly never completed without the help of competent and willing friends with expertise. I am very grateful to everyone who has supported me, not just with this book, but throughout my entire journey in crystals and healing. I want to thank everyone who believed in me and allowed me to "experiment" on them whenever I was given a procedure by my invisible tribe and trusting me to work on and with them with the multitude of layouts and healings that came through.

My gratitude goes to my friend, Patty Cauley, who suggested I see Rennie Laing to help heal my shoulder. I am so grateful to Rennie for not only helping me to heal, but to also assist me in opening my mind to the vastness of this Universe and the possibilities that it has to offer if we simply pay attention and listen.

Thanks to Marene Martensen, Joyce Hamm and Joan Collins for always being there when I needed them and for believing in me and my vision for Free Spirit Crystals. The foundation of our friendships has never wavered in the search for uncovering the truth and beauty in the world.

Thanks to Rose Koremenos for joining me at Free Spirit School and helping to expand beyond the genesis of an idea and into a full-fledged curriculum of healing with stones and crystals. Her inspiration and brilliance was and continues to be invaluable.

Special thanks to Michaela Wirtz for painstakingly and patiently editing this book knowing that I needed a calm and steady hand to walk me through the process. Once I write something, I loathe rewriting it and Michaela knew how to guide me through with the least amount of stress and pulling my hair out. This book would never have been completed without her.

And, to my invisible tribe, this whole crystal experience would never have happened had I not been hit in the head with a softball and awakened to the infinite possibilities in the Universe. I learned how to listen to the voices and trust in the wisdom of Universal energy. While I am the vessel through which this book was written, I am certainly not the creator of the healing techniques and layouts. I have been divinely guided these past thirty years and am humbled and filled with grace knowing that there is a power much greater than I showing me the way.

Acknowledgements

When I first started learning about healing with crystals and stones it was a very foreign concept to me. It seemed very esoteric and sometimes not very useful. Most of the books I read talked mostly about working with the Spiritual realm but not on how to connect the energy to the physical body. I knew that if I wanted to be an effective crystal healer, I would need to show people how the stones could be used in a practical way.

So, when I began to connect to the crystals, I experimented mostly on using them on the body to first prove to myself that this really worked. Even though I had healed my shoulder using stones, I still didn't feel like I had enough physical evidence of how to use them to for healing. My goal back in 1991 was to make crystal healing a practical modality so that more people would understand it and be able to use it on themselves and others.

This book is a compilation of my years of experimentation, listening to Spirit, everyday use, and hundreds of healing sessions to bring you a pragmatic approach to crystal and stone energy healing. It is my hope that you use this information and these techniques to improve your health, gain a clearer understanding about your life, obtain a greater sense of purpose and wake up to the magnificence that you possess.

Using this book

I'm a pretty practical person, which may sound strange considering the work that I do, but I felt that I needed to make this work more "down to earth" which is one of the reasons I wrote this book. My desire was to Keep It Simple Spirit and stick with the basics and a more step by step approach.

This book is a culmination of my thirty years of working with crystals and stones for healing. I developed a teaching curriculum from my experiences working with the minerals which is the basis for this book. I have included explanations about different types of crystals, the usage of stones for healing, explanations of the chakra system and levels of the field as well as various healing techniques.. There is an additional chapter on lists of stones for different healing situations that can be used as a reference.

Start at the very beginning and slowly work through the material. You will create a foundation for your own individual healing, as well as an understanding of what it takes to become a crystal healing practitioner.

I invite you to practice, practice, practice in order to develop your skills and knowledge. Open your heart and mind to new possibilities of being and becoming and trust that the Universe is the ultimate healer. I wish you well on this journey and hope that you find a way of life that is fulfilling, loving and blessed.

KISS GUIDE TO HEALING: HEALING IS FEELING!

Contents

Healing Techniques

Introduction

Sometimes the Universe Really Needs to Get Your Attention

If we're lucky, most of us will experience an unexpected event that will alter the course of our lives. Oftentimes, we sleepwalk through life without thinking about the ramifications of our thoughts and actions, or how we can make a difference in this world. Our motivations for life are instilled in us by our parents, teachers, friends, and institutions, and we strive to find security and happiness through the framework of our beliefs. But sometimes an event will occur that will force us out of the safety of our routines, and change our course in ways that we never imagined.

I was certain that my partner and I would amass our fortune, and eventually retire to travel the world, eat exotic foods and live out our days in a house on a lake. That's the course I had planned, and the plan was going very well until I hit the wall of dissatisfaction working in the corporate world. It seemed as if I woke up one day and nothing made sense. The bottom-line mentality hit me in the stomach like a sledge hammer. I just could not justify working to satisfy stockholders and CEO's. It was as if my conscience began to override my plans, and I knew I had to find something else to satisfy the longing that churned in my stomach.

In July of 1990, I decided to quit my job in corporate food service, and take a year off to search for a job that would bring more fulfillment. I loved the 'service' part of my job but the joy of that was being strained by the pressure of net profits. The problem was, I didn't know any other field except the one in which I was working, and I felt I had no direction.

Here's where it gets interesting! The day that I quit, I was pitching in a softball game, as I'd done hundreds of times before. I was quick on my feet and had great reflexes. I prided myself on my fielding and agility.

I never saw the line drive that hit me in the mouth, lifted me off of my feet, and landed me awkwardly on my right shoulder, causing a separation. Lying unconscious on the ground, my teammates thought that I was dead as it took me awhile to wake up. When I did, I saw the proverbial stars surrounding my head. Looking up into the night sky, I said to the Universe, "What?? What is this? I quit my job to explore my life and now I'm hurt? What the hell?"

With a swollen mouth and an arm dangling down my side, I was taken to the hospital where I began my education of our medical system. After a very painful x-ray, my arm was put in an uncomfortable harness.

A few days later, I found out that the harness had been put on upside down and backwards. The doctor gave me some pain pills and told me my arm would be fine in six weeks. Case closed!

After six weeks, not only was my shoulder not fine, it was worse. I was told to see a specialist. He could not determine what was wrong so he gave me a cortisone shot and ordered six weeks of physical therapy. The cortisone shot did absolutely nothing and neither did the physical therapy.

Six weeks later, I went back. He gave me another cortisone shot and six more weeks of therapy. As you can probably guess, neither one was effective. Every time I moved my arm it felt like I was being stabbed with a knife. No one knew what to do for me.

This went on until I visited the doctor the following June. He said that he thought that I had a pinched nerve in my shoulder – and he could do an operation to scrape away some bone and this would free up the nerve. Simple operation and I'd be fine. Not knowing any other medical model for healing besides allopathic medicine, I agreed to the operation.

All went well and the doc said I'd be playing softball again in six weeks. Six weeks – the magical time frame for healing! Needless to say, not only was I not better in six weeks, my shoulder was worse.

It was very discouraging. I couldn't use my arm. I couldn't work. I couldn't play. I couldn't even carry a bag of groceries. This was not what I expected when I quit my job to explore my life!

When I went back to the doctor one more time, hoping that he had come up with a new explanation and solution, I had a very eye-opening experience. He asked, "Now, which arm did I operate on?"

I thought he was kidding. When I realized he wasn't, it occurred to me (because I catch on a bit slowly) that there was a disconnect between what I thought our medical care should be and what it actually was. Doctors don't know everything. Sometimes they didn't seem to care, and sometimes healing actually had nothing to do with medical procedures and drugs. I declined another cortisone shot, which was the only solution he had left, and walked out of his office wondering how in the world I was going to heal my arm.

I decided to call my friend, Patty, who was a therapist, to see if she could recommend a different doctor. Instead, she suggested that I see a woman who did energy healing with crystals. What? Crystals? After I'd had the best therapy that Western medicine could offer, I should see someone who used rocks?

I thought this to be quite absurd and, when I questioned Patty's sanity, she asked, "So, what's your solution?" I realized I didn't have one.

So, I scheduled an appointment with the 'crystal healer' and started to learn that there was more to healing then I had been taught.

The healer, Rennie, had me lie on a massage table and placed stones on my body as well as in my hands. She did what she called Reiki healing and touched different energy centers in my body, explaining to me where I had energy blocks and having me describe my feelings. Describe my feelings? I'm German and Swedish! I didn't even know I had feelings!

But there I was, lying on her table loaded down with stones, checking in with my body and asking it to feel! Come on, this had to be some kind of a joke – except that it wasn't. I did begin to feel – anger, sadness, shame, fear – and it surprised me that I had all of that inside of me. Where was this coming from, and why had I not felt this before? Was she some kind of witch putting a feeling spell on me, hexing me into changing into somebody else? There had to be some kind of explanation for all of this!

At this point in my life, I did not have a spiritual compass. I had left the church a few years prior because religion just didn't make sense to me anymore. But I had not explored any other avenues or received any answers about what this Universe meant to me. I just wanted to make money, retire and travel!

But, when Rennie and the stones started shifting my perspective, I realized that there was something I was missing. The same dissatisfaction that propelled me to quit my job was now throwing me head long into a new life. I was dissatisfied with who I was, with who I'd become, with a void inside my heart that seemed too deep to heal.

The more I worked with the stones, the more I began to feel and, the more I began to feel, the more I was able to release the wounds and hurt of the past. I began to understand that healing had much more to do with the connection to our body, mind and spirit. A connection that, for the most part, Western medicine does not understand.

After working with Rennie for five weeks, I woke up one morning with no pain in my arm. It was like a miracle to wake up without pain. I decided to test it so I went into the pantry and found the heaviest thing I could lift – a case of soda! I lifted it over my head and had no pain! I did it several more times just to make sure this was real, and each time there was no pain.

My arm was healed, but even more importantly, my spirit was beginning to heal as well. I felt a great humility towards my life that I had never felt before, and a desire to find out everything that I could about energy healing.

Now, during the time my shoulder was injured, I began to hear voices. Not ever having heard voices in my mind before, I thought that perhaps being hit in the head had caused some form of mental disorder.

But the voices were very loving. They didn't ask me to do harm to myself or anyone else. They just wanted to talk to me about life. Mostly the voices came to me between 3:00 and 3:30 a.m. which was really pretty annoying because I needed all the beauty sleep that I could get!

The messages I received were interesting and nothing like I'd ever experienced before. I was being questioned about my happiness, the level of joy in my life, who did I believe myself to be – you know, easy stuff!

So, I listened, not really understanding where all of this was leading. I do believe now, that when I got hit in the head, it aligned my crown chakra antennae to the Universal internet, and I was downloading from a cosmic Wikipedia!

I did question whether these voices were coming from my own head, or if they were really my invisible spirit guides. Once, when they woke me up at 3:00 a.m., I told them to leave me alone because I was not in the mood for a pre-dawn chat. I gave them a problem that I had been grappling with and asked for a solution. They told me to look in a certain book and gave me the specific page number and paragraph, which I wrote down, and promptly fell back to sleep. The next day I found the book, page and paragraph and there it was – the answer to my dilemma! Could I have made that up?

Another time, I was lying on the bed pretending to do a meditation because they had told me to meditate! I had no idea what that was so I faked it. The voices came to me and I said to them, "So, if I'm not making you up, give me the dimension of this room."

The answer came back immediately: 16 feet. Well, I know the room was not 16 feet wide so I got a tape measure and measured – for whom I do not know – 14 feet. "Aha!" I said, "I am making you up. This room is 14 feet wide!"

I instantly heard from my invisible friends, "Not if you measure diagonally," So I measured the room diagonally and, sure as termites love wood, it was 16 feet wide! Alright, they had me. I was convinced that I was not hallucinating. I wasn't fabricating voices. I actually had some kind of channel connection to the ethers. How interesting!

A few weeks after my shoulder was healed, I was lying in bed with my partner, watching Murphy Brown. This is one of those times when you remember exactly where you were, what time it was, and what you were doing. My friendly spirits talked to me as clearly as if they were sitting next to me and said, "It's time to start your crystal business now." Plain and simple – start a crystal business now. The end of conversation!

Well, I was beyond flabbergasted that this was the message du jour because I knew nothing about crystals, other than they had helped to heal my arm. I knew nothing about the healing properties of crystals and stones. I had little money because I had not worked in over a year. I didn't want to open a store and have that kind of responsibility. It just didn't make sense that they would want me to represent them doing this type of work.

So, I said, "No." But, being the persistent buggers that they were, they insisted that this was what I was supposed to do. In my head I argued with them, giving them every argument that I could think of to not to agree to this proposition. I have a business degree. I knew that you did not start a business not truly understanding your product, not having at least 3 – 5 years of capital to keep you going, not having a customer base, and not having a business plan to take to the bank!

But, every time that I gave them a reason why I couldn't do this, they gave me the solution as to how I could.

Don't want a store? No problem – you're going to set up tables at flea markets, spirit fairs, county fairs, anyplace that people gathered to buy things. Problem solved!

No overhead? Problem solved!

Don't have much money? You don't need a lot. Find a place to buy some stones and set up a table in your spare bedroom to display them. Problem solved!

Don't know your product? We'll send you a teacher. Problem solved!

Business plan that I need to get a business loan? This is it, I thought! No bank needed. Problem solved!

Still not being convinced that this was a good idea, I asked them, "Why do you want me? Why not find someone who already knows about the stones, knows about healing, knows how to use them? Why pick someone who obviously knows nothing?"

Their answer was clear and to the point: "Because we need someone who will sell them at a reasonable cost so that more people can have access to them. And, we know that you will do that. We trust you."

Well, I had no idea about the profit margins of stones, and I didn't really much care because this was such a lark to me. I started laughing out loud and my partner turned and asked, "What's so funny?"

So, I explained to her the message that I just received and she started laughing. "What are you supposed to call yourself? Pick and Save Crystals? Crystals R Us? Get Your Bargain Crystals Here?"

It did seem absurd and so I decided not to make a decision until the next day. I told them I'd get back to them.

The next day I called my friend, Patty, and told her what had transpired the night before. Her immediate reaction was, "Absolutely! Do it!" Really? You're a therapist. Aren't you supposed to give me guidelines and words of caution?

So, I called my healer, Rennie, and told her the same thing. She had the very same reaction as Patty. Just do it! I explained that the problem was that I didn't know anything about crystals and stones. She told me to come on over and she would show me. There was my teacher!

Then, I told her I didn't know where to buy stones. She told me to go to Mount Ida, Arkansas because that's where the crystals were. There was my source! She said she would price the stones for me so that I could start selling them and gave me suggestions as to where I could set up a booth. Easy, easy, easy.

Needless to say, I agreed to the Universe's terms and started Free Spirit Crystals in September 1991. Their 'business plan' turned out to be exactly what I was looking for in my life. I was working for the best bosses possible; I was doing a service that I loved, I was helping others and I found the joy in life that had evaded me.

Without my wonderful 'cosmic wake-up call,' I would not have discovered the most important aspect of my life – me! Getting hit in the head was the best thing that ever happened to me. It woke me up to the endless possibilities that the Universe has to offer and allowed me to become the person I always wanted to become. Free Spirit Crystals has been, and continues to be, a vibrant cog in this community for people to discover their own selves, to wake up to their own lives and dreams.

I will be forever grateful for that not so soft ball smacking me in the face and allowing me to find a Universal calling. This work is my passion, my soul purpose and it fills my life with joy. May you find that for your life in whatever way you are called to do it.

Healing Basics

Chapter One

Healing Naturally

It's important to note that when you start to use crystals and stones, your life will change. Not might change or could change, but will change. This energy works not only on the physical level, but on the emotional, mental, and spiritual levels as well. One level does not function without the other, and thus it is called Holistic Healing or Whole-Istic Healing. If we want to heal ourselves, we need to heal all aspects of our lives. That is true healing.

There may come a time in your life when nothing seems to be working, nothing seems to make sense, nothing is the same as it used to be, and nothing seems to help. Understanding that life is more than what you have been taught to believe, that true healing comes from within, and that each of us is responsible for our own healing is the awakening that we all must realize on our path to a whole existence.

This healing modality allows us the gift of shifting our way of life, understanding the relationship between our ancestral background and the pattern of our lives, assists in changing our belief systems, understanding how and why we feel about ourselves, the relationship between the self and spirit, and the gifts that we each possess and need to claim in order to fulfill our lives. We each come into this life with a purpose. And, it is through our evolution that we claim our purpose and use our lives as stepping stones towards becoming whole.

How Quartz Crystals Work

Let's begin with the basics. Quartz crystals are composed of silicon dioxide (SiO2). Silicon dioxide is comprised of two oxygen atoms and one silicon atom connected molecule to molecule, locking and interlocking in a spiral growth pattern. As the crystal grows, a mathematically precise and orderly lattice of atoms is formed into a grid-like structure. This interwoven arrangement is highly geometric and has a spiraling energy pattern. Think of the DNA helix.

Crystals form in the ground through a combination of water, heat and pressure. Researchers have discovered that quartz crystals have a unique ability to convert electrical energy to mechanical energy and vice versa. This is called the piezoelectricity (pahy-ee-zoh-i-lek-TRIS-i-tee) effect. In 1880, scientists Jacque and Pierre Curie first demonstrated that this effect, ultimately creating the foundations of the quartz technology revolution. Silicon is the basis of the semiconductor industry.

The Curies proved that quartz had the ability to receive, process and transmit precise vibrations which stimulate energy in many forms of technology. The crystalline structure of quartz responds to heat, light, pressure, sound, electricity, gamma rays, microwaves, bioelectricity and even energies of consciousness.

Computers, digital watches, radios, sonar, electric guitars, electrical units in cars, satellites, oscillators in precision instruments such as optical lenses in medical and surgical equipment, all operate on crystalline energy.

The U.S. military made the decision to incorporate crystal controls into all of its communication systems in 1939. Military historians say this decision greatly contributed to the Allied victory in World War II.

An early use of this resonance was in phonograph pickups, where the mechanical movement of the stylus in the groove generates a proportional electrical voltage by creating stress within a crystal.

Today, a crystal oscillator is a common piezoelectric use for quartz. The vibration frequency of the crystal is used to generate an electrical signal of very precise frequency.

The Quartz Connection to Our Body

Fascinatingly, our bodies also have a silicon base. It has been shown that the pineal gland, which some consider to be the master gland, is made up of crystalline compounds. Our bodies are composed of an electrical system known as the nervous system and, when crystals are used on the body, they assist in aligning the master gland with the nervous system. Quartz is said to have the closest vibration to the human body of any other mineral, giving it the ability to balance our energy systems.

Human beings are fully immersed in energy. Most of the things in, around, above and below us have measurable energy – some are tangible, some are not. Within our bodies we have the invisible energy forms of pain, thoughts, emotions and knowing. Around us we have harnessed ultraviolet, infrared, electricity, sound waves, microwaves. We breathe oxygen and give off carbon dioxide. This is all energy.

And, like all of these things, quartz crystals are filled with energy and represent an energetic modality to balance and align us physical, emotionally and spiritually. Quartz can also help to clear our energy fields of the EMFs that pervade our lives, helping to dispel their effects on our bodies. Quartz crystals represent an energetic modality to balance and align us physically, emotionally and spiritually. All of the qualities of quartz, combined with our own consciousness, contribute to the well-being of our body, mind and spirit.

The Energy of Stones

Everything in the Universe is energy. Everything is made of up atoms, neutrons, and protons – and all of the other things I didn't pay attention to in high school science class. Energy is continually moving. You can feel it in the wind, in the vibration of a train going past, in the touch of a hand. There is vibrational energy that is more difficult to sense – touching a car door, a piece of furniture or a wall. But these things are still vibrating; they are still in motion.

Having grown in the earth for thousands, and sometimes millions of years, gives every stone its own unique vibration and individual consciousness. When different stones are placed on the body, it aids in shifting the energy blocks that we develop over the years.

One of my teachers told us once that 'everybody's got something' and we need assistance in healing that something. Nature had given us these minerals to assist us in bringing our bodies back into its natural alignment. This process allows us to connect to different levels of our energy field, including the spiritual, mental, emotional and physical. The stones not only bring energy into the body, but also emit a vibration that reaches out to the other three levels, helping us to heal the whole.

When I was in the process of healing my shoulder, I began to have emotional feelings and mental realizations of things that had happened to me in my life which I'd never experienced before. I began to understand that I was hanging on so dearly to the life I thought I was supposed to have, that I was preventing myself from moving into the life I was meant to live.

When I fully got that concept, the pain in my shoulder was gone. I had freed myself up and given myself permission to move forward, to leave the past behind and to explore the new me. It was a complete body, mind, emotion and physical healing. The consciousness of the crystals and stones worked on the blockages of each level in order to make the healing complete.

The earth has given us great gifts. Ancient cultures understood the value of the earth's treasures – stones, herbs, oils, foods – and cultivated their healing aspects. But, somewhere along the way and, for many reasons, we forgot or neglected to bring it forward into the modern era.

We are rediscovering these natural remedies and incorporating them into allopathic medicine. We do not need to choose one or the other – both can be used in harmony with the other. When I was diagnosed with stage 4 lymphoma, I chose to use allopathic medicine, but I also used my crystals and stones, meditated, journaled and ate a healthy diet in order to heal quickly and thoroughly.

According to Western medicine, curing an illness or injury means alleviating the symptoms. It doesn't necessarily include addressing the underlying cause. However, a complete healing needs to include getting to the crux of why we got sick in the first place.

Up to 90% of illness is stress-related. Well, what if we could do something to not have that stress in the first place, or are able to deal with that stress in natural ways that actually helps us fully heal?

I believe that crystals and stones bring this type of healing to us. It's all nature, it's all energy, and our bodies are energy systems that fall out of alignment. When we can bring that alignment back, we can heal ourselves. But it takes determination, dedication and a new way (or old way!) of looking at things to make it happen.

Now, I would never suggest not seeking medical help if you need it. I go to the doctor on a regular basis, and have needed some of the drugs prescribed to control illness in my body. However, we can use the stones, crystals, herbs, oils and healthy food to make our healing a complete experience. Healing is about letting go of the past, letting go of old belief systems and patterns that no longer suit us, forgiveness, and becoming the person that we truly want to be. Everyone can heal – but the cure might not be what you think it should be!

It is my own opinion that, because quartz has the ability to retain information, it holds records of the eons that it has been in the earth. We can access that information through meditation and channeling. We can also program crystals to assist us with whatever issue we are personally working on. I have done this many times with great success.

<u>Uses for Quartz</u>

Structure and Balance	Transmits energy
Amplification	Aids in communication
Stores Information	Enhances and enlivens psychic abilities
Brings focus	Clear and activates chakras
Transforms energy	Resolves emotional disturbances
Purification	Energizes the levels of the field
Energizes the physical body	Bring harmony and perfection
Aids in meditation	Relieves pain
Aids in concentration	Assists in healing
Cancels harmful effects of radiation and radioactivity	Brings mental clarity

Chapter Two

Guidelines for Crystal Healing

I experimented a lot with stones and crystals when I first started. I discovered that there were basic principles that can be useful in doing healing work. These guidelines are helpful for knowing which stone to use for certain situations, for keeping the work simple and practical, and to help gain confidence in yourself when you are beginning to learn. If you learn these simple guidelines, you can begin working on yourself today!

One of the easiest ways to start is to do a simple stone layout on yourself. This will allow you to begin feeling the energy of the stones throughout your body. While it is best to have the stones directly on the skin, it's not always possible to do, especially when you're in a group or if you are doing a session on someone else. Placing them on your clothing is still effective as the energy is capable of sifting through fabric.

By knowing the colors of the chakras, you can match stones of these colors to the chakras to do a layout for balancing and clearing.

Colors of each chakra:

First Chakra – Red or Black

Second Chakra – Orange

Third Chakra – Yellow

Fourth Chakra – Pink or Green

Fifth Chakra – Light Blue

Sixth Chakra – Dark Blue or Violet

Seventh Chakra – Violet or Clear (White)

Choose whichever stones you wish for your layout as long as they are these colors. My favorite basic layout is:

First Chakra – Black Tourmaline

Second Chakra – Carnelian

Third Chakra – Citrine

Fourth Chakra – Rose Quartz

Fifth Chakra – Sodalite

Sixth Chakra – Amethyst

Seventh Chakra – Quartz Crystal

This is a layout that will begin your process of acclimating to the stones and allow you to have a relaxing experience. I recommend doing this for 20 minutes, once a day, for one week. I encourage people to journal after each session; to write about their feelings and experiences in order to learn how their bodies shift after time.

It's important to note that, although all rocks appear to be hard, some are softer than others and have different uses. In 1812, a German geologist named Frederic Mohs defined the hardness of minerals on a scale of $1 - 10$. Although mostly used in manufacturing, I have found the Mohs scale to be helpful in ascertaining which stones are used for drawing out energy blockages and inflammation, and which are good for permeating into the body to aid in releasing energy impediments. My assessment is that stones from $1 - 5$ assist in drawing out from the body, and stones from $6 - 10$ penetrate into the body.

Soft and Hard Stones

Soft stones draw out negativity and heavy energy. Hard stones penetrate into the body to assist in breaking up energy blockages. Soft stones are useful in relieving inflammation and releasing blocked cellular memory. Harder stones are used for unlocking deep seated core issues in order to move forward in life.

Terminated Stones

Stones with terminations, or points, direct energy up and down through the point. Drawing a terminated stone clockwise over the body directs energy inward. Drawing counterclockwise draws out negativity, heavy energy and blockages.

I invite you to take a crystal point and move it in a circular motion about an inch from the palm of your hand. Notice what you're feeling – tingling, heat, movement.

Crystals are electromagnetic and, when used on the body, they connect with our own electromagnetic field. The direction of the circle one draws over the body will determine whether the energy is being drawn out or penetrating in.

If you wish to draw out negativity or inflammation, draw counterclockwise on the area. This lifts out the energy impediment. By drawing clockwise over the area, you will direct energy into the blockage to assist in breaking it up.

I will sometimes try both to ascertain which is most effective for the situation. The more you work with the crystals, the easier it will become to determine which method to use. With enough experience, the stone will tell you what is needed.

Smooth Stones

Smooth, flatter stones permeate outward and down into the body. Imagine that you have dropped a stone into a pond. Watch the water as the stone drops and the ripples move outward. Placing smooth stones on the body have the same effect. These stones cover a wider area and assist the body in moving more energy and releasing more blockages.

Striated Stones

Striated stones have grooves that run up and down the surface of the mineral. Energy in these stones will move in the direction of the striations in order to remove stagnant energy from between the chakras, and to open clogged energy in the meridians. These stones work quickly and directly which is quite different than smooth stones which permeate into the body.

Examples of striated stones include Selenite, Tourmaline, and Kunzite.

25

<u>Energy Flow</u>

Holding stones in the hands or placing them on the soles of the feet allows the energy to flow throughout the entire nervous system.

All of the nerve endings in our body are connected to the palms of our hands and the bottoms of our feet. When we hold a stone in our hands, the energy will release itself throughout our body. This will help in regulating our nervous system, balancing our energy and utilizing the purpose of whichever stone you are using.

Every stone has specific healing attributes so when you choose a stone to hold, those aspects will flow through your physical body and your consciousness. I invite you to choose a stone to hold in your hand and to simply allow yourself to feel what is happening. The more you sit with the stones, the more acclimated you will become with feeling the energy.

Note: Even if you do not 'feel' anything happening, it is! Everyone feels things differently – there is no one way to feel the energy. But nature dictates that everything is vibrating and everything has energy. When we hold the stones in our hands or place them on our bodies, that energy will move through you. Electricity will move through you, heat moves through you, sound moves through you – and so does the energy of stones and crystals. It's simple!

26

Chapter Three

Clearing and Cleansing Crystals and Stones

Because minerals consist of vibrations, they can absorb and transmit energy. We do not know what environment the stones were in before they came to us, so it is important to clear each one before we use them. I clear my stones before and after I use them on others, as I do not want another person's energy to affect the next client I work on. Even when I use the stones myself, I clear them because they are picking up and clearing things inside of me. I want them to be as energetically pure as possible the next time I use them.

I learned a good example of how crystals hold on to another person's energies from a friend of mine. She had gone to see a crystal healer and, as she was lying on the table, her back began to hurt. She looked under the table and noticed a huge crystal point beneath her. She asked the woman when was the last time she had cleared the crystal. The woman replied that she did not need to clear it.

Needless to say, my friend got up and left. We always need to clear our stones before and after we use them. I cannot stress that enough!

Here are a few ways that I clear my stones:

Light Invocation

In the first crystal class I took, I learned DaEl Walker's crystal healing techniques. DaEl had the innate ability to simplify working with crystals, and his methods were so practical that I love his work. He believed that using crystals should be functional. He experimented to come up with the most useful clearing technique.

Here is his method for clearing crystals and stones: hold them in your hand and say the Light Invocation three times:

I invoke the light of Universal Energy within.

I am a clear and perfect channel.

Light is my guide.

I use this technique every time I work with stones. You can hold several in your hand at once to expedite the process or put them in a basket, place your hands over them, and say the invocation above the stones. You can say the invocation in your mind making this an unobtrusive technique. Do this before and after you use them. When working with a client, you may not always have a sink available to rinse your stones so this technique is an efficient method to use when doing a session.

Sunlight

Stones love the natural cleansing energy of the sun. The light and heat purify them and leave them with sparkling energy!

One word of caution with placing stones in the sun, however. There are certain stones that you do not want to keep in the sun for long periods of time as the color will fade from them. Examples include: Amethyst, Fluorite, Celestite and Kunzite. You can expose them for short periods of time, but not for more than a few hours.

Moonlight

If you have a window ledge where the moonlight enters or a safe place to lay your stones outside, the full moon offers a lovely way to clear and cleanse them. The indirect light from the sun will assist in bringing back their luminosity without fading them.

Rain or a body of water

Stones love to be showered with natural water (sans chlorine or chemicals) so placing them out in the rain is very cleansing. I also have rinsed them in rivers, lakes and the ocean. If you do this, please make certain that you secure them – I learned this the hard way and lost a couple of my favorite stones in the current! Placing them in a mesh bag and tying it tightly is a sound idea!

One word of caution – there are a few soft stones that should not go into water as they will eventually dissolve or break apart. Be careful with Selenite, Hanksite, Pyrite Suns, or any stone with a 1 or 2 hardness on the Mohs scale.

Cold, running water

If my stones become very heavy and sticky, I will run them under cold tap water. This removes the outer grime and releases any inner negativity that they may have picked up. If I am using my crystals on a client that has a lot of issues, I oftentimes find it necessary to use this technique in order to continue. It makes the crystals feel clean and refreshed.

Lukewarm water with Joy® dishwashing liquid

If you have a lot of stones that are sitting around on shelves or in baskets, you can place them all in a tub and wash them all at the same time. Stones don't have egos so they don't mind taking a bath together! I like to use Joy® dishwashing liquid simply because I like the name! Be certain to rinse them well when you are finished to remove soap residue. For an extra treat, you can place them all in the sun to air dry!

Smudging

You can use sage, sweet grass or your favorite incense to smudge your stones. You can devise your own ritual around this by saying a blessing at the same time if you'd like. You can also sage your healing space or sacred meditation room doing the same thing.

<u>Sand</u>

If your stones feel like they need an extra shot of energy, you can place them in a pot of sand or soil. This is their natural habitat and a little boost of nature's ground can help revive them. Just remember where you plant them!

<u>Salt</u>

Some people will place their stones in sea salt but this is not my preferred way. I find salt to be too abrasive for the crystals and, because there are so many other ways to clear them, I like to avoid the salt technique. However, if you find this to be effective, do use it. There are many who think this is a perfectly fine way to clear stones.

Last thought: sometimes the stones will simply wear out. They will 'feel' done. In that case, thank them, bless them and place them in your garden or bury them in the ground. They have done their job for you!

Crystal Basics

Chapter Four

Crystal Identification

Crystals and stones have been used since the beginning of mankind as healing agents, talisman, meditation tools and prophecy oracles. We may have forgotten the wisdom of the people who came before us, but now is the time for rediscovering what our ancestors learned long ago.

When I first started my crystal business, I knew absolutely nothing about crystals, how they were formed, what they did or how to use them. I thought each one was cut in a factory to form the shapes until I made my first trip to the crystal mine in Arkansas. As I stepped out of our van, I found a perfectly clear tabby teacher crystal at my feet. I was so excited that I yelled to whoever was listening that crystals grew this way naturally! I'm sure they must have looked at me like I fell off the mountain and hit my head because no one seemed very impressed at my discovery! But for me it was a day of awakening that began a life-long study of these amazing treasures.

There are many different natural formations on crystals that make each one unique. Here are most common ones that I use in my own practice.

Cathedral Lightbrary

A Cathedral Lightbrary is distinguishable by the growth of crystals attached to the core crystal and cascading upward. Most of the base will be encased by crystals growing around most or all of it. These stones are hard to find but if you do manage to get one, it will be a very personal stone for you.

I first saw a Cathedral Lightbrary when I was studying with Katrina Raphaell in Hawaii. She had one in her house on a pedestal which she brought out for us to do a group meditation with. It was about a foot tall and adorned by beautiful crystals around the entire core. The energy radiating from it pulsed out to the group, and made it easy for us to enter a meditative state. I'm surprised the roof stayed on her house after we were done!

A Cathedral Lightbrary can be used to access your pages from the Akashic Records and to attain inner wisdom.

Alice A. Bailey's description of the Akashic Records still resonates: "The Akashic Record is like an immense photographic film, registering all the desires and earth experiences of our planet. Those who perceive it will see pictured thereon: The life experiences of every human being since time began, the reactions to experience of the entire animal kingdom, the aggregation of the thought-forms of a karmic nature (based on desire) of every human unit throughout time." [1]

Accessing your Akashic Records can assist you in understanding your spiritual evolution, the lessons that you have learned and continue to learn, and how you can

---

[1] [1]Bailey, Alice A. (1927) Light of the Soul on The Yoga Sutras of Patanjali

use these lessons to attain nirvana.

This crystal assists in accessing group relationship information and is also used to attain innate inner wisdom. We all access information that we simply know – we don't know how we know it, it's just there for us. The Cathedral Lightbrary allows us to develop more of that knowing so that we can bring more of our truth to living this life.

Channeling Crystal

The first crystal I ever owned was a channeling crystal. I had just learned how to use a pendulum and discovered that I could use a Channeler to access information from what I call the "Intergalactical Information Highway." Some people claim to communicate with spirit guides, angels, ascended masters and master teachers. I like to think they're all on the IIH.

A channeling crystal has a front with seven facets and, directly behind that, is a triangle. Seven is the number of spiritual searching, gathering information, and study while the number three is the body, mind, spirit connection and communication. When they are on the face of a crystal, they combine to assist us with transferring messages telepathically.

My business went through a very rough time during the early 2000 recession. I didn't have the money to spend on lots of advertising and I really needed to reach more people besides through social media. So, I used my channeling crystal to ask my guides exactly what I could do to keep Free Spirit Crystals afloat.

Within a half an hour I was given very specific instructions how to proceed. Now, I didn't really like what they told me because it forced me to get out of my comfort zone. I was told to contact other metaphysical businesses to ask if they would be interested in having me present free crystal healing workshops for their customers. I am not the most outgoing person in the world so, for me, venturing out into unknown arenas was a very uncomfortable suggestion.

However, I did ask and they did offer a solution so I did exactly as they said. Within a few weeks I had several offers and was able to reach many more people who became not just good customers, but great friends. I was able to sustain my business until the economy turned around, and also learned some valuable lessons about allowing myself to be seen!

Sometimes it takes a while to connect with the "Intergalactical Information Highway." I used to sit at my kitchen table for hours with my crystal and a pendulum until I was able to feel comfortable that I was truly communicating properly and with ethical guides. There are what I call 'the tricksters' who will come through just to play with you. You can tell them apart from your guides because the information will sound silly or not of use to you. Just remember to be discerning and check in with yourself to make sure what you're getting sounds logical and safe.

To practice, you can hold the channeling crystal in your left hand with the point facing the wrist (the left side of your body is typically the receiving side), have an intention or question that you would like clarity with and simply wait until you 'hear' an answer.

You can also hold a pendulum over the crystal and ask yes or no questions to start the process. There are very good books available on how to use the pendulum and, if you want to use this tool, I suggest that you read one and practice. Trust that what you are hearing is from your guides and that you are not making it up. Or, you can test them like I did to verify that what you are getting is the real deal.

A channeling crystal can be used to gain a connection with your own guides, angels, teachers, etc. It can be used in a grid with the Channeler in the middle and an array of other stones placed around it in a circle. This intensifies the energy of the channeling crystal and amplifies the power of the communication.

This crystal also helps us to access our own inner thoughts and inner spirit. Remember, our pineal gland is made up of crystalline compounds so using a Channeler also opens us to our own information. It can help us to progress spiritually by clarifying our purpose in this lifetime and providing guidance as to how we may proceed with our lives in the most spiritual manner.

<u>Crystal Cluster</u>

You can identify a cluster because there will be a number of crystals growing our of the same base. A cluster can be as few as two crystal points up to thousands of crystals. Each point on a cluster emits a line of light which helps to clear the environment of negativity. If you have a room in your house that feels heavy or dark, placing a clear quartz cluster or two in the window or in the corners of the room will assist in transmuting the energy into a more positive tone.

I have a fifty pound clear quartz cluster with over a thousand points on it which I keep in my living room. When people come into my home, they almost always remark about how light and happy it feels.

My partner worked as an operation's manager for a world-wide company and faced many challenges everyday with employees and management. I gave her a nice crystal cluster to place on her desk so that, when negative people came into her office, it would help keep the atmosphere more positive. After a couple of months on her desk, the crystal became very cloudy as it had absorbed the negativity from those who came into her office and prevented that negativity from affecting her

In the '90s, I lived in a beautiful old Victorian house that had lots of history in its bones. The living room was stunning with a large fireplace, huge bay windows, original decorative plaster moldings and a twelve-foot ceiling, but no one wanted to sit in there. Everyone congregated in an add-on room at the other side of the house. I was determined to make the living room hospitable so I took crystal clusters and placed them all over the room, on the fireplace mantel and in the bay windows. Within a few weeks, people started to congregate in the room and it became party central.

Crystal clusters absorb negative energy from your environment and transmute it into positive energy. It also helps to clear other stones. Just place the stones directly on the cluster.

You can use it for manifesting by programming it with your intentions for the higher good. It opens the crown chakra to help communication with guides. And, it's a great tool for group meditation.

Devic Temple

Devic Temples have ledges inside of them caused by infractions or cracks within the crystal. These ledges are said to house earth sprites and fairies.

These crystals remind us to lighten up and to have a more childlike nature. They can display impressions of other worlds, temples, or faces and outlines of beings inside and, thus, are useful for scrying and divination.

They also help to transform one's attitude to gain a more positive outlook on life. And, they can help us to communicate with sprites and fairies to learn what they have to teach us.

Double-Terminated

Double-terminated crystals have points on both ends of the stone, allowing the energy to move back and forth or through the crystal to transmute negative energy.

I place double-terminated crystals in between the stones placed on each chakra when I do crystal sessions on clients. This helps to expedite the movement of the energy up and down the entire chakra system. I find it to be a very effective method to energize sluggishness and promote vitality in the body.

I have also used double-terminated crystals to help me learn while I sleep. I place the crystal with one point next to whatever information I want to remember and the other point facing my head. Of course, I have to also read the material before I do that, but this helps me to retain the data.

My friend, Marge, told me that she had difficulty remembering her dreams. I gave her my 4-inch double terminated crystal and an elestial crystal. I instructed her to place the Elestial on her nightstand with one point of the double terminated crystal facing it and the other point facing her head. She did this for several nights until her dreams became vivid.

Double-terminated crystals take in energy, purify it and transmit it through the other end. They are excellent for astral projection and dreaming.

They can provide protection from mental and physical harm by helping us to maintain a strong energy field. These crystals also help to open and strengthen our psychic abilities.

<u>Dow Crystal</u>

Dow crystals are said to be the "crystal of perfection." Discovered by Jane Ann Dow, these stones have three channeling faces and three triangles in between them, thereby cubing the energy of a channeling crystal. They help to promote balance in one's life and enhance spirituality.

I like to use a dow crystal when I want to clear my mind and get a more direct line of communication with Spirit. With the power of three channeling crystals on board, I find it easier to start the process of connection.

A Dow attunes you to the 'perfection of God Energy.' It enables you to acquire knowledge from both the Universe and from within your own being. And, the Dow will assist you in expressing your intent and in communicating with all realms of creation.

Great for meditation and focus, it brings the perfection of the Divine into one's consciousness to assist in perfecting one's life.

<u>Elestial Crystal</u>

Elestials can be identified by their chunky, scaly looking exterior, unlike their hexagonal cousins. They are sometimes known as Jacaré or alligator skin quartz, making them very recognizable.

My first experience with an Elestial was in the fall of 1992 when my partner and I went crystal mining in Arkansas. After getting our fill at the mines, we decided to scour the countryside for places to buy stones. We happened upon a man who had a private collection and invited us to buy some of his pieces. I spied a particularly odd-looking crystal, smoky in color and craggy exterior. He explained that it was an Elestial that he had mined himself in the hills near his house but that he was reluctant to sell it. He must have noticed the droopy, puppy eyed look I gave him and he agreed to part with it.

I slept with my new treasure and noticed that I was receiving information in the middle of the night. It was mostly about my past and what I needed to do to move forward – perfect for that time in my life. I realized that this crystal held intelligence of the eons, and that it could help us with understanding the patterns of our lifetimes in order to heal the present. I have dubbed the Elestial the "Grandmother/Father" stone as it holds generational knowledge for us to access.

Elestials are the gift of the angels. They hold the treasure of wisdom and knowledge from the beginning of all time. You can access answers to questions on any level of your being, that of Mother Earth, or the Universe.

This also crystal assists in overcoming emotional burdens. It brings the emotions and intellect into synchronicity. It helps us to feel our feelings and to find self-love. Elestials are sometimes called the "Enchanted Crystal" as it brings a feeling of newness into our life after each phase of growth. It helps us to prepare for transformation, the release of control, and can assist with our journey to enlightenment. Coupled with a double terminated crystal, it also helps with lucid dreaming.

Fadens

The word faden is German for thread and these crystals have a gaseous line running through them that look like thread. They are usually flat crystals, although I have seen some that are hexagonal. Fadens are mainly used for connecting lines of energy either on the body for healing or for telepathic communication. They are particularly useful when used as a bonding agent to heal the physical body in the form of broken bones, or mending cuts and scrapes.

Fadens are also effective when used for communication in relationships. They are said help to strengthen the bond between those in conflict, bringing in clarity and truth.

I like using faden quartz on the body when I do sessions because it is flat and won't roll off, and because it helps to connect the energy between chakras. I place them in between the chakra stones with the thread pointing to the stones for the best connection and energy movement.

Fadens are also conduits for energy thoughtforms and healing. They connect one energy to another and help to open blocked passageways. They are useful for physical healing and are good meditation tools as they open channels to higher knowledge.

Gateways

Gateway crystals are laser-like, in that they are very slender crystals with three very narrow sides with three sides wider and flat. These six sides make up a sphinxlike face on one or more of the sides. When you look into any of the three wide, flat sides of the crystal, there are spaces at the top that are defined as gateways. On the backside of the sphinxlike face, the gateway goes through the face of the crystals into what is described as the next or other dimension.

When I studied with Katrina Raphaell in Hawaii, I took a trip to Hanalei Bay on the north side of the island. There, I found a wonderful little place called Avanna's Goddess Shop and met the owners, Avanna and Robert. They had an assortment of items promoting goddess energy and, in the back, they had a few stones. When I told them that I was in Katrina's class, they asked if I would like to see the shipment of crystals that had just come in. The stones were still in the boxes so I had the thrill of unpacking them – it's like Christmas for me – and examining all the crystals.

There was one crystal that I could not identify so I asked them if I could take it with me to meditate with that night. They were happy to let me do so because I also offered to identify and price their entire shipment of crystals. Now, that's what I call a vacation! At any rate, I meditated with the stone and asked it what its name was. I immediately heard "Gateway." I'd never heard of a Gateway so I asked what it was used for, and how I could use it, which I journaled.

The next day, I showed it to Katrina and asked her what kind of crystal it was. She replied that she'd never seen one like it and I thought, "Oh boy, I've discovered a new crystal shape! I'm going to be a famous crystalogist!" As you can see, the ego can still get in the way even when doing spiritual work!

I showed the crystal to several class members and asked them to sit with it and find out its name. They all came back with some form of Gateway – Gate Keeper, Keeper of Light, Way of Light, etc. I decided to keep the name it had given me because I had been the one to discover it.

I went back to Avanna's and found a few more Gateways that I purchased and brought home with me. I will be forever grateful to Avanna and Robert for their generosity and openness.

When I returned from Hawaii, I was idly flipping through Love Is in the Earth: A Kaleidoscope of Crystals, by Melody, and I came upon a passage that talked about a gateway crystal. I was dejected to know that I had not been the one to discover it, but also elated because it had told me what it was and some of the information that I had gleaned from it was in Melody's book. It was a confirmation that I truly was tapping into the great stone encyclopedia in the sky and that I was not making it up.

At any rate, I was told was that the Gateway is the stone of truth. It is a taskmaster that will hold you accountable for staying on the straight and narrow, ethical path. It is a stone that assists in learning about your reason for being in this lifetime, the lessons you need to learn, and how to learn them.

It's a wonderful stone for communication either between people or cosmic energies as it is very direct and to the point. There is no interference in the wires when using a Gateway.

One technique that I learned from the Gateway was how to clear the mind. One night, I was holding two gateway crystals and had the urge to spin them. I held the crystals in front of me, points facing each other, and started twirling the crystals around each other. I could feel a build-up of energy and then, after 15 – 30 seconds, I stopped and placed a crystal on each temple with the points facing my head. I felt an intense buzzing, immediately followed by a line of energy going through my head from one crystal to the other, giving me an instant clarity of my mind.

I learned to take the crystals off after no more than ten seconds, however, because otherwise I got dizzy with a mild headache. It was a great lesson in the powerful energy that crystals can both generate and transfer.

Gateway crystals assist in our evolution. They provide a higher harmonic vibration that enables you to learn about your contract, life patterns and your purpose of being. Other crystals can be used to access past lives and give information about your path and your Soul's purpose, but this particular crystal can help you to receive this higher knowledge concisely and clearly, removing any cobwebs that may still be in the way. As conduits of truth, gateway crystals temper the information received from previous lives, and tie this knowledge together into an understandable progression from one lifetime to next.

Gateways may be used to open mental gateways between individuals for better communication in their relationships. They provide mental clarity on your path forward.

Generators

You can tell a Generator from the other crystals because all of its equally sized facets meet directly at the tip of the crystal. Whereas other crystals may have 3 – 5 lines meet at the top, the generator has all six and this creates a very focused and direct energy.

They are very powerful crystals for generating positive energy. Generators can be used to change your environment by programming them with an intent for whatever you wish.

I had a three-pound generator that I used in a meditation class. We programmed the crystal with a group intention, then placed 12 crystals around it, each facing outward, to amplify the energy of the programming. Each week we would meditate around the crystal to concentrate on our intent.

Generator crystals can be used on an individual level or through a group effort.

These crystals cleanse chakras and replace negativity with radiant, white light. You can place a generator under your healing table to expedite the power of a session. But, remember – these crystals magnify energy and must be cleaned after every use!

Isis

This crystal is named after the Goddess, Isis. In Egyptian mythology Osiris, Isis' husband, was chopped up into tiny pieces by his jealous brother, Seth, and strewn throughout the heavens. Distraught, Isis turned into a bird and gathered up the pieces of Osiris' body to bring him back to wholeness.

You can recognize the Isis crystal by the 5-facet face on at least one side of the crystal. Symbolically, the two short lines that frame the base represent the soul's foray into the physical dimension, allowing us to experience all of our physical senses. The two longer lines that meet at the tip embody our unified reality while the two opposing lines signify contradictory forces.

The focal point in this crystal helps to bring back to us all of our scatter parts – our childhood traumas, our broken hearts, our conflictions and judgements about ourselves – in order to become whole. This is a wonderful stone for emotional and spiritual healing.

Isis is used for balancing dualities and to bring polarities together. They support keeping us centered so that we do not go too far to either extreme. They assist us in understanding the need to make changes in our live and support our ability to allow these changes to integrate into wholeness. And, this crystal assists the soul to enjoy life and to truly learn about the physical plane.

Keys

A key crystal has an indentation in one of its sides. This indentation can be anywhere from three- to six-sided. When I first saw a key crystal, I thought that the indentation was caused by miners poking into the veins of crystals with a hexagonal pole! It was only later that I realized this was a natural formation for the stone.

The indentation is said to unlock information that we all hold within ourselves. The cells of our body hold the memory of everything we have experienced in our lives. Key crystals assist us in lifting out that information because we hold the key to all of the answers that we need to find about ourselves. The 'key' is to look inward, not outward, for fulfillment and happiness.

You can put your thumb on the key and meditate with it, or you can use a pendulum to gain information from the crystal. Just remember, you are responsible for yourself and hold the solutions to all of your questions and inner obstacles.

These crystals can help unlock inner mysteries, act as doors to healing concepts, and assist in analytical problem solving.

Laser Wands

Laser wands are generally rugged looking crystals that are tapered from the base to the tip. This makes the energy very focused and very fast.

These crystals are useful for building a shield of protective light around an object or person. To do this, walk around the person or object while pointing the crystal outward. I do this around my car before I take a trip or around my house if I feel any negativity in my area.

I once used this technique when I wanted to buy a house. This particular house had several offers on it but I really, really wanted to own it. So, while I was 'inspecting' the property, I took out my laser wand and walked around the house three times chanting, "This is my house, this is my house." That night I got a phone call with the good news that my offer was accepted.

Another technique you can use if you feel negativity inside your home is to walk around each room facing the laser wand towards the walls and saying a blessing for the room. This puts a line of protective light in the space. You can also do this to cleanse your meditation or healing room.

I use laser wands to do auric 'surgery,' an advanced healing technique that assists in removing blockages and unwanted energy from the seven levels of the aura. Before attempting this however, you should become well-versed in the levels of the field and strengthen your subtle sense perception. Although I have included information on the auric field, I recommend that you also study the chapters on the levels of the field from Barbara Brennan's book Hands of Light or find a competent crystal class or energy healing class that teaches this hands-on.

This book includes information on how to use laser wands to run lines of light through the body to open meridians, and how to do spine balancing using laser wands. Please read these chapters before attempting to use lasers on the physical body.

Important note: unless you are well-versed in how to use a laser wand for healing, do not point it at anyone as the laser wand's energy can cut through the aura. Much like a medical laser, this focused energy is very direct and sharp.

Manifestation Crystal

Manifestation crystals have one or more quartz crystals growing inside the main stone. These crystals remind us that the Universe has ample abundance for everyone and that the greatest abundance we have is inside of ourselves. Using this crystal as a meditation tool aids in finding the places inside yourself that are blocking your ability to manifest.

We learn from an early age whether or not we are worthy of receiving what we desire. Often this can grow into a belief that we do not deserve things. And so, we sabotage our efforts to manifest our desires, either subtly or overtly.

In my family of origin, we were taught not to be better than anyone else. That the meek would inherit the earth. That if you strove for something better than your family already had, you were showing off.

These beliefs became a part of my cellular structure and it took time and awareness to free me from my family's core teachings. The manifestation crystal helped me break those patterns and establish healthier ideas about who I am and what I can have.

Whether you want material things, a new relationship, a better relationship with yourself, or a new job, it is important to believe that you deserve to have it. I spent a great part of my earlier life hiding behind the belief of lack. It wasn't until I became aware of the conditioning that was holding me back, that I could step into my own self and ask for what I wanted. I didn't have to play small any longer!

<u>Masks</u>

When you look at a mask crystal, you see that there are two similar and yet different facets next to each other on the crystal's face. These facets are divided by vertical line, creating an almost mirror image of each other.

It's as if you look at your own face in a mirror. It may seem as though both sides of your face look the same. But, if you put the side of your hand up to your nose and visually separate each side, they may look very different. In this way, our face is the mask that we show the world and each day we put on a different mask, depending upon who we will see, where we will go, and what we will do.

Mask crystals ask you to look behind that façade and discover who is really inside of you. It begs the question, "Do you like what you see behind the mask? Are you happy with who you are? What are you hiding from yourself and the world?"

This crystal propels us to take an inventory of those things we do not approve of, or would like to change. In so doing, it asks us to take off the mask and emerge from the shadow to become our own light. And, it helps us to be honest with ourselves in order to live with integrity.

<u>Phantoms</u>

If you gaze into the depths of a phantom crystal, you will see a cloudy, ghost-like shape of a smaller crystal within it. Sometimes, this is very distinctive. Other times, it may only be a wispy and elusive outline. Phantoms are useful for connecting to, and understanding, our past lives and the patterns that we bring from lifetime to lifetime, in order to shift our consciousness and move on. They are especially helpful in working through family issues rooted in past beliefs and outdated loyalties.

There are several types of Phantoms, including Clear Quartz, Smoky Quartz, Amethyst and Chlorite Quartz. Clear Quartz connects well with our subconscious mind. Smoky Quartz works well with issues of the family. Amethyst is useful for connection to the spiritual realm. Chlorite is wonderful for cleansing the physical body as well as our thoughts.

This crystal can help you find your missing parts and integrate this knowledge into your wholeness on all levels of your being. It can assist in bringing us clear and positive ways of thinking.

<u>Rainbows</u>

Rainbow crystals are formed by inclusions or internal cracks within the crystal. A prism forms in these infractions, causing lovely rainbows to shine through. These rainbows represent joy, love, and bliss. They help connect us to those aspects inside of ourselves.

They help to connect us to Universal Love and remind us that we are not separate beings but a part of the 'All.' Rainbow crystals are calming, reminding us to not take life so seriously, and to embrace our inner child.

Rainbows have a heightened energy flow and help us to become more balanced. They support emotional healing by helping us release sorrow, lightening our hearts and our minds. Place one on your heart and allow yourself to feel what you are afraid to feel and let it go!

Record-Keepers

Record-keepers are crystals that have a raised or embedded triangle in one or more of the crystal's facets. Sometimes, they are quite small and you really have to search for them. Other times they are quite pronounced and immediately recognizable. It looks like the triangle is etched right on the face of the crystal.

On occasion, record-keepers will develop on a crystal after you have had it for a while. This has actually happened to me and I know that there is information that the crystal was holding just for me.

Record-keepers are very personal crystals. If you are drawn to one, there are very specific messages waiting for you to access. I find them to be quite chatty once you are able to open yourself up to listening to the messages. I like to hold the record-keeper in my non-dominant hand and then place a pendulum in my dominant hand to organically swing over the crystal and start the line of communication. I 'hear' the messages and write down or record what I'm hearing so that I retain the information. It is a stone I use when I need a question answered or am feeling stuck in a situation and need a strategy to help me out.

If you don't immediately get answers, don't give up. You can also meditate with them, place them under your pillow when you're sleeping, place them on top of a piece of paper with your questions on it or place it in a grid that you devise for a specific intention.

Record-keepers are crystals in which ancient knowledge and wisdom, from the civilizations of Lemuria and Atlantis, have been stored. The information encoded in the crystals is for your personal development or for the betterment of Mother Earth.

These crystals also assist with developing or enhancing your psychic abilities – clairvoyance, clairaudience and clairsentience. Keep practicing every day until these abilities become natural to you.

Remember, the number three – as represented in the record-keeper triangles – is the perfect balance. And, record-keeper crystals can assist us in bringing that balance into our lives.

<u>Rutilated</u>

Rutilated crystals have lines of titanium dioxide growing inside of them. These filaments of iron oxide can be anywhere on the color spectrum from red to gold, to silver to black, depending on the iron oxide content. It's easy to recognize this crystal because it will look like it has little needles of metal growing on the inside.

Rutilated Quartz is a powerful mineral as the metal filaments help to intensify the energy of the stone. It goes deep into our energy field to access the most hidden emotions and blockages, allowing us to become aware of what we have hidden inside of ourselves. It's a powerful stone for shifting cellular memory and drawing in positive energies for emotional, mental and physical healing.

Rutilated Quartz's powerful energy enhances our ability to go beyond 'normal' thinking in an effort to understand that everything is possible. It helps us to get out of our own way in order to transform thoughts, ideas and beliefs.

This crystal also supports learning channeling, astral projection, scrying, and connecting to astral beings. This transformational tool is ready when you are!

Self-Healed

Self-healed crystals are the only crystals that you can identify by looking at the bottom of the crystal. These stones broke off from their matrix while growing and then repaired themselves by forming a cascade of tiny, crystalline triangles on their base. This symbolizes our ability to continue our own growth, even when life interrupts.

There are times when it all seems too challenging to keep going. Self-healed crystal reminds us that being broken is a temporary state and that we can continue to grow through perseverance and faith. Just as the crystal takes a break from its continued growth, we can do the same. The test is to have the courage and strength to start again, and renew our devotion to shifting and growth.

This crystal gently gives us courage to move forward in our spiritual growth and in finding forgiveness, both for ourselves and others. This helps heal the emotional, mental and spiritual wounds and move forward with new courage and conviction. If you are stuck in such a rut, get yourself a self-healed crystal and let it show you the way.

<u>Tabby</u>

Tabby crystals are flat 6-sided crystals that look like something very heavy sat on them. I like to use tabby crystals because you can place them on the body and they won't roll off – very practical! Tabby crystals are great for connecting one chakra to the other. If you place stones on each chakra and a tabby crystal in between each one, it helps to move the energy of the stones up and down the system for a lovely chakra balancing.

Tabby crystals can be used to enhance telepathy between two or more individuals or between you and your spirit guides/angels, etc. It also is a great crystal for clearing the mind of clutter to make decision making easier and to alleviate confusion.

Tabby crystals are great connectors. Use this crystal to activate other crystals and stones. It also supports mental clarity.

<u>Tantric Twin</u>

Early on in my crystal journey, I was having a challenging time in my long-term relationship. So, I laid down on the bed with a Tantric Twin and asked my guides to show me what a healthy relationship looked like. They said, "Clasp your hands together but don't let your arms touch. This is your relationship. If one of you takes their hand away, the other is dangling, and not knowing what to do without the other. Neither of you has a strong enough sense of your own individual lives to feel whole without the other.

"Now, clasp your hands and bring your arms together. You can unclasp your hands and there is a base by which you can relate because you both come to this relationship strong in your own self. This is a healthy relationship. You can come together and go apart and still have the stability you need in a relationship."

Well, I thought that was quite brilliant! If you look at a tantric twin crystal, there is one solid, secure base with two individual crystals on it. Without that solid base, they would fall apart. This teaches us to work on our own lives in order to bring a whole person into a relationship. We cannot rely on another person to make us happy or bring us what we need. We are each responsible for our own happiness. But, with two people who understand that, relationships have the roots and stability to stay together.

You can also use Tantric Twins for working on group dynamics, to help people understand their roles and how to relate to each other in a healthy manner. Awareness of who we are is always the key to any relationship!

These crystals help us to perceive information about relationships on all levels of our being, and to facilitate in the building of our relationships on all levels. Tantric Twins bring the understanding that love brings freedom. And, this crystal unites the consciousness of groups.

Time Links

Time link crystals have a distinct parallelogram that forms a window on one or more facets. If the parallelogram tilts to the left, it is said to connect to your soul's past. If it tilts to the right, it connects to your soul's future. Sometimes, a crystal will have both a left and right time link window. This connects us to the current moment.

This crystal serves as a bridge between your Higher Self and your soul's experience. You can work with a Time Link to access information in order to gain a higher understanding to help heal old wounds, or to bridge the gap between past lives. This gives us a broader perspective of our soul's journey and insight as to what still needs to be learned.

Since time really has no structure other than what we give it, it is possible to suspend our beliefs about time, and to access any point on the spectrum that we desire. What would you like to know about your past lives? What issues did you bring with you into this life that you still need to heal? What do you need to understand that will bring you peace of mind and allow you to move on? These are all questions that a time link crystal can assist with.

Transmitters

Transmitters have a perfect triangle at the center of the crystal with two symmetrical, seven-sided facets on each side. Transmitters do exactly what their name says – transmit energy and information. Because they have two seven-sided facets, they are ideal for gathering information from other dimensions. They are also very useful for accessing the Akashic Records and for contacting your guides.

Transmitters are ideal for long-distance and absentee healing because they send energy wherever you program them to. You can place them on the picture of someone who requests healing by lovingly programming the person's name into the crystal with whatever healing intention he/she needs. You can, if you wish, say a blessing or the Light Invocation into the crystal to enhance the energy. You can also do this for group healing or by using Reiki energy along with it.

These crystals can be used to talk with spirit guides, especially if they are trans-channelers. I like to use my pendulum as it assists in getting the energy flowing, and supports a nice, clear connection. The more you practice this, the stronger your telepathy and clairaudience will become.

Transmitters are also helpful in healing your personal life as these crystals assist us in the application of universal knowledge and wisdom into your consciousness..

<u>Windows</u>

A window crystal has a small and distinct diamond shape where the sides of two facets meet, usually between the main body and tip. Most are found in clear quartz points, but you may also find this shape in Citrine or Amethyst. These crystals are often hard to find, so if you have the opportunity to get one, snap it up!

Window crystals are said to open a window to your soul. If you want to understand your reason for being here, why you are going through the challenges that you are experiencing, what you need to learn in this lifetime, and what you need to heal, this is one of the best crystals that I know of to use. It brings clarity to your thinking, helping to pop the illusions of the world and brings a clear vision of reality.

A Window will come to a person when he/she is willing to look honestly at themselves and are ready to do the work. The information you are given may not be what you want to hear, but what you need to hear. You will gain spiritual courage and a deep sense of who you are in relation to the Universe. Be ready to cut through the nonsense and get to work!

This crystal helps you to see clearly that which you hide from yourself. They can help us move outside of our own comfort zone and examine the uncomfortable places inside. It can help us examine the interim between lifetimes to assist us to truly understand the lessons to be learned in the present lifetime.

Chapter Five

Chakra Basics with Stones

In this chapter, we will walk our way up the seven main chakras and discuss the healing aspects of over fifty stones. This information will give you a basic understanding of the chakra system, which stones correspond with each chakra and how to use them.

Muladhara – Root Support
Color – Red
Element – Earth
Sense – Smell
Physical Location – Base of Spine in
Tailbone Area

First Chakra

The root chakra governs life lessons involving the material world, such as survival, and stores information involving family beliefs and loyalty, your ability to stand up for yourself, superstition, instincts, physical pain or pleasure, and touch. Your sense of self-esteem, safety and security are also based here. Feel the need for fight or flight kick in? Thanks to a connection to the adrenal cortex, your root chakra just activated!

This chakra is related to our survival instincts, sense of grounding and connection to our bodies and the physical plane. It anchors the body physically to supply the life force we need and it holds our genetic inheritance for vitality and innate predisposition to disease.

The root chakra is connected to our adrenal cortex as this stores our inherited ancestral energies. It sends energy into our bones, spine, sacrum, nervous system, our blood, sexual organs, and our legs, hips and feet.

When blocked, or restricted, it creates a lack of life-force throughout our body. Disease/unbalance can lead to physical issues such as anemia, heart disease, high blood pressure, sexual and gynecological disfunction, autoimmune deficiency, drug addiction and even cancer.

Emotional Imbalance: Loss of interest in the 'real world' and practical survival, obsessions and addictions, volatile emotions, selfishness, restlessness and a lack of energy.

Excessive Energy: Egoistic, domineering, greedy, sadistic, or sexual energy focused entirely in the genitals.

Deficient Energy: Lack of confidence, weak, can't achieve goals, suicidal, a feeling of being unlovable, low interest in sex.

Imbalance Energy: Inability to stand up for oneself, fear, a sense of not belonging or victimization, attachment to material things, eating disorders.

Balanced Energy: Strong sense of self, centered, grounded, healthy, fully alive, unlimited physical energy, can manifest abundance

How to rebalance our first chakra: Slow deep sound that resonates into the pelvic floor, tailbone and lower spine, sleep, eating a well-balanced, nutritional diet, grounding exercises and/or yoga poses, working on family/security issues.

Mantra: I have the right to be.

<u>Crystals/Stones:</u>

Although the suggested color for the root chakra is red, I like to use a lot of black stones here. My other rule for crystal/stone healing is to throw out all the other rules and go with what you feel and with what works for you.

Black Kyanite: Black Kyanite is a fan-shaped stone. The bottom point helps to draw in scattered root chakra energy. I find it very useful for grounding and centering.

I like to place a Black Kyanite on each thigh with the point facing up towards the second chakra. This placement is best for bringing the earth energy up into the root and aligning the chakra. I have used this technique on people who have been diagnosed with bi-polar disorder to help them stay centered.

Black Obsidian: Black Obsidian is another very hard stone. Native Americans call this the "Shadow Stone" as it helps us to see our shadow side. I use this stone when a client has hidden some uncomfortable truths from themselves and the world around them.

In order to heal on an emotional and spiritual level, we need to be aware of the clouds that veil the truth. Black Obsidian helps to crack the shell of our resistance.

A word of caution when working with this stone– don't use too much too soon! It can actually cause the body to shed too much at once, resulting in nausea and body aches. Deep healing needs to be done gradually so that we are able to assimilate the information and emotions that occur.

Black Obsidian is also useful in helping to break addictions because, when we understand why we have an addictive behavior, we can shift the energy of that behavior towards a healthier lifestyle.

Black Onyx: Black Onyx draws out memories from the root chakra to guide emotional and spiritual healing. It helps to absorb negativity and purify the chakra system. It also assists in dealing with grief and anxiety. Sometimes, I will use Black Onyx on someone after I have had them use Black Obsidian as it helps to temper the effects of the Obsidian.

Black Tourmaline: Black Tourmaline is a very hard, striated stone that I call the "Rotor Rooter" because its energy spirals up through the chakra system to help 'clean out' the blocks and imbalances and to align the chakras. I like to place this stone in between the knees rather than directly on the root chakra because I like the flow of energy it produces up and down the legs as well as up to the other chakras.

Black Tourmaline is a wonderful grounding stone which also assists in centering the body. It aids in safeguarding one from outside negativity.

Hematite: Hematite is the best grounding stone that I know of. Its iron base causes it to be very heavy, which allows us to stay fully connected with our body. It helps with memory and concentration as it brings scattered mental energy down to the root chakra and centers it.

Hematite is also said to be effective in strengthening the circulatory system and aligning the spine.

Pyrite: Although Pyrite is a golden color, I have found it to be a wonderful root chakra stone. Its weight assists with grounding and its color works to deflect negative energies. It helps to increase stamina and give our body more vitality. It can actually be used on all the chakras.

Pyrite is also known as the "Traveler's Stone" as it is said to protect people who take trips. My advice: keep one in your car or your suitcase.

Smoky Quartz: Smoky Quartz has been naturally radiated in the ground which gives it different shades of brown. It is also is a hard stone whose energy penetrates deeply into the cells, allowing the erosion of energy blocks. Smoky Quartz is a calming stone that helps to alleviate trauma events that impact our root chakra so that we can fully integrate our healing in a calm fashion. Smoky Quartz assists in dealing with family issues and physical survival.

Svadhishthana – Sweetness
Color – Orange
Element – Water
Sense – Taste
Physical Location – 1-2 inches below
the navel

Second Chakra

The sacral chakra is about friendliness, creativity, sexuality, intimacy, emotions and intuition, manifestation and interpersonal relationships. It is connected to flow of first chakra. Beliefs embedded in the first charka extend 'branches' into the second. Our sacral chakra holds these connections to tribe, culture and community. It stores our duality, magnetism, controlling patterns, and emotional feelings.

This chakra relates to our sense of self-worth and our confidence in our ability to create. This is where our 'gut-level' intuition operates from. It supports our ability to connect with others in a friendly and personable way. And, this chakra governs our sexuality, especially for women, and enables healthy sexual relations.

Physically, the second chakra is linked to our skin, kidneys, spleen, the middle of our spine and female reproduction organs.

When this chakra is not in balance, we may feel the need for emotional protection from those who are toxic in our lives. Low self-confidence or a lack of motivation may manifest due to feelings of self-criticism, imminent failure and a general disappointment in what we have been able to accomplish in our life.

Unbalanced Physical: Low back pain, sciatica, ob/gyn problems, pelvic pain, libido, urinary problems.

Unbalanced Emotional: The need for power and control, a lack of morality, aggressive, manipulative, self-indulgent, emotionally explosive, distrustful, overly sensitive, immobilized by fear, shy, overly sensitive, hard on self, abused, loss of creativity, feeling guilty about or obsessed with sex.

Balanced Energy: Optimistic, belonging, creative, intuitive, attuned to feelings, sense of humor, sexually in tune.

How to rebalance our sacral chakra: Identify and heal emotional upheavals, balancing the feminine, healing family issues, exercises/yoga for hips and lower abdomen.

Mantra: I love and enjoy my body.

<u>Crystals/Stones</u>:

Bloodstone: Bloodstone is a great stone to help boost the immune system and aids in clearing blood infections, bladder, liver and kidney maladies.

In 1992, after my shoulder was healed, I decided that I needed to see a therapist because I'd heard that if you have parents, you need therapy. So, I went to see a wonderful woman named Marge Rock (I chose her because of her last name!).

I recently had gotten in a shipment of stones and there was one particularly beautiful Bloodstone that I placed in my pocket, determined to keep it for myself. As soon as I placed it in my pocket, I heard it say, "Give me to Marge." I had an appointment to see her that day but how did the stone know that? At any rate, I said no. I wanted it and that was that.

So, it said, "You have to give me to Marge." Have to? That sounded like a challenge so, again, I again no! Well, that stone would not let up and kept hounding me!

I went to my session that day. As soon as I walked in, Marge said that she was sorry but she had a severe bladder infection and would need to reschedule our appointment. I took out that gorgeous Bloodstone, handed it to her, and told her that she needed to have it.

When she asked me why, I said that I just had a feeling. I wasn't going to tell a therapist that stones were talking to me! She thanked me and advised that she was going to see a doctor later in the day.

That night, she called me. She said that, by the time she saw the doctor, the bleeding and the pain had stopped. Did I think it was the stone that helped? Well, of course I did, but I said to her that I wasn't sure but it may have.

So, just an FYI, when you are ready to do this work, the Universe will continue to give you proof that it really works!

Carnelian: Carnelian is a great stone in promoting creativity, and building the energy needed to start and complete projects. It supports promoting your talents and aids in building confidence. It is helpful for digestion, gently opens the sexual centers, and aids the circulatory system. It is also good for helping to alleviate lower back pain by helping us work through our personal security issues.

I had a client with lower back pain who placed a Carnelian on her bed stand when she slept. One night, she woke up with a burning sensation in her hand and found she was holding the Carnelian. She placed it back on the night stand and woke up, again, with the Carnelian in her hand. The next morning, her lower back pain was gone. Everyone has different issues and different timelines for healing, and this was a wonderful example of how Carnelian works.

Moonstone: Moonstone has feminine energy and works with the phases of the moon to assist with our body's cycles. It is great for alleviating menstrual pain and the mood swings associated with menopause. One time I had gotten my period but didn't have any aspirin in the house, so I grabbed a handful of moonstones and placed them on my belly. The cramps went away.

I thought I might be making this up so I took them off. The pain came back so I put them back and the pain went away. I did this several times just to test it and the results were always the same. From then on when I got my period, I simply put Moonstones in my pockets and never took pain medication again for my cycle.

Moonstone also helps to regulate our emotions and keep us on a more even keel. This stone is helpful for both men and women when they feel overwhelmed by pent up anger or frustration because it helps to balance the male/female energy ratio in the body.

Moss Agate: Moss Agate is a lovely green stone interspersed with white Chalcedony. It actually looks like there is moss in the stone. This is a wonderful stone for clearing toxins, cleansing the blood stream, and healing infections. I place a washed Moss Agate on cuts and abrasions to assist in the healing process.

Moss Agate is useful for long-term illnesses, and to assist and strengthen the immune system. It works well with kidneys and the liver.

Red Jasper: Red Jasper helps to bring vibrancy and endurance to the body and is wonderful for strengthening the organs such as the liver and kidneys.

This stone enhances our feelings of personal power and independence, and can help with overcoming shyness. This is a very determined stone. It guides us to focus on what we really need, and not just what we want. It helps remove negativity in our thoughts and actions in order to build a more positive attitude.

Ruby: I call Rubies the "Hot Stuff" stone as they help to fire up the second chakra and get us moving. It is a demanding stone and will not take no for an answer. So, if you decide to use a Ruby, please note that you will be strongly encouraged to put your gifts and talents to immediate use. If you don't, you will feel edgy and incomplete until you are motivated to begin what you are meant to do. I have a two-pound Ruby sitting next to me right now as I write this book so that I keep on task and finish it!

Rubies also enhance sexuality and sensuality. I've had many women buy them for their husbands and boyfriends!

A word of caution: Rubies can help release pent up anger. This is great for people who have difficulty expressing themselves, but not as helpful for those who prone to anger.

Third Chakra

Manipura – Jewel City
Color – Yellow
Element – Fire
Sense – Feelings
Physical Location – Solar Plexus

The solar plexus chakra governs the will, the mind and our emotions. This chakra is about digestion at a 'gut' level, both assimilation of nutrients and digestion of thoughts.

This chakra is a powerful will center and the source of our vital energies. Located just above our navel up to the sternum, it is here where we connect to our own personal power, recognize our accomplishments, and feel a sense freedom to truly be ourselves. This where our clarity of thought, increased awareness, and curiosity are located.

We experience a connection with our psychic experiences with the third chakra. There is a direct relationship between our ability to project our will into manifestation and this chakra.

This center is constantly challenged in humanity. An imbalanced or overactive charka may manifest as becoming judgmental, demanding, stubborn, extremely emotional, of always planning but never doing.

Many of us are taught from early childhood to repress our emotions and feelings. Repression of emotions can cause you to lose touch with your feelings and this can become a danger to your life force.

Our stomach, upper digestive tract, pancreas, liver, gall bladder and diaphragm are physically linked to our solar plexus chakra.

Physical Imbalance: Anxiety and fear, digestive problems, heartburn, reflux, ulcers, pancreatitis, appendicitis.

Emotional Imbalance: Judgmental, demanding, stubborn, emotional in the extreme, perfectionism, procrastination.

Out of Balance: Powerlessness, greed, doubt, anger, and guilt, excessive worrying.

Underactive Energy: Depression, lacking in confidence, worrying about what others think, afraid to be alone, self-pity, confusion, poor digestion, fear of failure, apathy, feeling isolated.

Balanced Energy: Outgoing, cheerful, open and expressive, intelligent, self-confident, flexible, respect for self and others, ability to express feelings.

Mantra: I love and accept myself.

<u>Crystals/Stones:</u>

Amber: Amber is fossilized tree resin and is very soft. It helps uncover deeply buried issues to help you love and respect yourself. It draws negativity out of our bodies and transmutes it into positive energy. Used as a talisman, Amber provides protection from psychic attacks and outside negativity.

I worked with a few men who contracted AIDS and I meditated on what stone I should give them. I was told to give them Amber because all of them had very low self-esteem and felt an incredible amount of shame for having gotten AIDS. I had them place the Amber on their solar plexus and allow the energy to assist them in processing their emotions. We all discovered that there can be a great healing without being cured of a specific disease.

Citrine: Citrine is known as the "Stone of Manifestation" but, rather than simply giving us 'stuff,' it helps us to recognize what our fears are around feeling worthy. We all have beliefs of what it is to have 'enough' and when those beliefs limit us, we have difficulty allowing ourselves to have what we want and need.

Citrine is the best stone that I know of to help us work on fear issues. I call it the "Fear Buster." When I first started using stones, I realized that my life was filled with fear and, that in order to become my true self, I had to understand what was holding me back. I would sleep with a Citrine sphere in each hand at night and, when I awoke each morning, I would journal what I had experienced in my dreams or what feelings has arisen. This journal helped me to understand the genesis of my fears, to realize that fear is something that is taught, and that Citrine is a , with awareness, fear can lessen or be alleviated.

Citrine is a wonderful stone to help build self-esteem and confidence. It encourages us to be more outgoing and present our true self to the world. Who would you be if you had no fear?

Lepidolite: Lepidolite is another stone that I use on the solar plexus chakra even though it is purple. Its natural lithium content assists in calming anxiety and working with depression. It stimulates the feeling of self-love and self-acceptance and I find that the solar plexus chakra is a natural placement for these issues.

I like to place mica lepidolite underneath the adrenal glands to help boost the energy to combat adrenal fatigue. Sometimes when clients come in tense and anxious, I will give them a mica lepidolite 'bath' by placing pieces all over their body. The lithium content assists in relaxing the body and mind. Holding a piece of lepidolite in each hand helps the calming energy to move through the nervous system and provides rest and encourages sleep. It assists in releasing negativity to promote a more positive outlook.

Malachite: Even though Malachite is green, I like to use it on the solar plexus chakra. It's one of my rules – throw out all the other rules! We hold a lot of issues in our third chakra and, being a relatively soft stone, malachite helps in drawing out and releasing those issues. Malachite is a stone that is useful for using all over the body.

Malachite stimulates cellular memory to unlock stagnant feelings and emotional patterns. It is extremely helpful in reducing swelling - arthritis, bursitis, sprains, strains, etc.

My favorite example of using malachite happened one night in a beginning crystal class that I was giving. One of the students, Rose, came in late, limping. When I asked her why she was limping, she said that right before she came to class, she took her dog for a walk. As soon as they stepped outside, the dog saw a squirrel and took off after it, pulling Rose down the stoop and causing her to hit her heel hard on the pavement. I gave her a large piece of Malachite to rest her foot on.

Of course, she questioned my reasoning because she didn't really want to be in the class. She was enrolled in a different healing course but had missed the crystal class and was told to take mine. Being a medical professional, she thought crystal healing was woo-woo and wanted no part of it!

Ten minutes later her heel was becoming very warm and achy. Rose was certain that I didn't know what I was doing, but I told her to keep the stone where it was. After about twenty minutes she noticed that she no longer had pain in her heel and began walking around without a limp.

Needless to say, she was convinced of the healing nature of stones and we now run The Free Spirit School of Integrated Energy Healing together! Plus, she uses stones in her healing practice and with her animals.

Tiger Eye: Tiger Eye is a stone for self-confidence and believing in yourself. It helps to give us a backbone so that we can stand on our own two feet and trust ourselves. It helps us to tune into our 'gut' feeling and to know what is right for who we are. It gives us the courage to act on our ambitions and dreams and to assimilate thoughts and ideas in order to act on them.

This is a lovely protection stone from unwanted interactions and negative environments. I like to give this stone to children who are shy and unsure of themselves or to those who are bullied. It encourages them to be themselves and have a more harmonious outlook on their lives.

	Anahata – Unhurt, Unstuck
	Color – Green
	Element – Air
Fourth Chakra	Sense – Touch
	Physical Location – Center of Chest

The heart chakra is concerned with love and the connection between our physical bodies and our spiritual selves. It is the midpoint of our consciousness and our physical bodies. It lies halfway between the three lower chakras, which are aligned with keeping us moving in the physical realm, and the three upper chakras, which keep us growing in the spiritual realm. I call it the Grand Central Station of the chakras.

The heart chakra is also the midpoint in our spiritual bodies. It lies halfway between Mother Earth, who is our connection to the physical plane, and Father Sky, who is our connection to the spiritual plane. Balance lies in the recognition and acceptance that love is all there is.

When the heart is balanced, metaphysically every thought, word and deed will be undertaken in love. That love will be a force on both the physical and the spiritual planes. In that respect, nothing we think or do can ever be totally self-centered. We have a connection to others, and to ourselves, that supports an understanding and generosity in all aspects of our lives.

When this chakra is closed or out of balance, we may feel indecisive and afraid of letting go. We may fear betrayal. Or, we may feel unworthy of love and be in constant need of reassurance.

Physically, our heart, circulatory system, lungs, immune system and our endocrine system are associated with the fourth chakra.

Physical Imbalance: Difficulty breathing, pulmonary afflictions, circulatory afflictions, immune disorders, breast cancer, high or low blood pressure, allergies, upper back and shoulder issues.

Emotional Imbalance: Guilt, rejection, jealousy, self-pity, paranoia, unable to love yourself or others, hatred, indecisive, fear of letting go, fear of betrayal, the need for constant reassurance, melodrama, the use of money and sex to control people, a martyr complex.

Balanced Energy: Compassion, generosity, honesty, self-respect, healthy relationships, empathy, being in touch with feelings, the ability to express appropriate feelings of love, self- acceptance and acceptance of others, unconditional love, giving of yourself without expectation of receiving anything in return.

How to rebalance our heart chakra: Learn how to really live in the moment to heal your past, practice self-acceptance, focus on positive thinking and affirmations, connect with nature, work on forgiveness, declare a gratitude day, become a volunteer.

Mantra: I am open to love.

<u>Crystals/Stones</u>:

Aventurine: I call Aventurine "Adventure Green" because it takes a journey through your body to find energy blocks, and then stays in the area to help release them. I use this when I'm not sure where someone needs assistance, and often place it in their hands where the nervous system can take the energy throughout the body. It helps in unlocking unresolved issues and old beliefs and conditioning as it penetrates into the cellular memory and unlocks it.

Aventurine acts as a harmonizing agent and is said to attract good fortune and abundance. It promotes feelings of joy and helps to fulfill dreams.

Chrysoprase: Chrysoprase is a premier calming stone for the heart, and is ideal for those who have high stress lifestyles and careers. It promotes peace for the heart and acceptance of self and others. Chrysoprase assists with depression and anxiety as well as helping to lower high blood pressure in some cases.

I had a friend who worked 60 hours per week and had two children after the age of forty. Needless to say, her blood pressure was off the charts! I had a Chrysoprase necklace made for her and, after wearing it for a couple of months, her stress level had become manageable and her blood pressure was much lower. During this time, she learned how to delegate and give herself more time to be alone. Sometimes the stones are a reminder that we need to take care of ourselves!

Chrysoprase also helps to promote joy and love while giving us the awareness that we need to forgive in order to be truly happy.

Kunzite: Kunzite is a hard, striated stone with a lithium base giving it a calm, soothing presence. I call Kunzite the "Love Stone of the 21st Century" as it helps you to love and appreciate yourself and your own goodness. It assists in tapping into your magnificence and alleviates the judgmental voices in your own mind. By doing this, you make yourself more receptive to other's love and desire for you.

Kunzite helps as a calming agent in times of stress. Lie down on your bed and place a piece of Kunzite on your heart for relaxation and to soothe agitation. It is useful for those who anger easily or live in a state of irritation.

Rhodochrosite: Lovely Rhodochrosite connects our crown chakra to our heart chakra bringing down lightness and joy to our heart. It is a reminder to not take yourself so seriously, that life is meant to be enjoyed, and to give yourself a break from the outer world so that you can enjoy your inner world.

It is the stone of compassion. Rhodochrosite brings blissful love into our beings to connect our inner spirit with the Universal Spirit. It stimulates the dream state, thereby stimulating your sense of personal power. It works with the circulatory system to help regulate and stabilize blood pressure. It also helps to alleviate migraine headaches.

This stone connects our heart chakra with our crown chakra, allowing Universal love to enter. It helps us balances our emotions and promotes joy.

Rhodonite: Rhodonite is a pink and black stone that helps to connect our heart to our root chakra to ground and center the heart chakra energy. In connecting to the root chakra, it allows us to release the wounds of the past by using heart energy to understand and have compassion for ourselves and others. It is a wonderful heart stone for trauma and for releasing resentment and anger.

I like to use Rhodonite as a communication agent between couples in order to understand relationships. Each person carries a Rhodochrosite during the day and then at night exchange each other's stone and hold it. The energy of the stone will help you relate to what your partner's day was like, and assist in establishing an open line of communication. Talk about what your feeling as you hold the stone while keeping your heart chakra connected to your partner. The grounding energy of the Rhodochrosite will allow for a more peaceful and smooth conversation.

Rose Quartz: I call Rose Quartz the "Grandmother Stone" because it has a loving, sweet energy that says, "Come here and let me rock you. You're fine just as you are." It exudes a soft, accepting vibration that allows us to be comfortable and relax.

Rose Quartz is known as the relationship stone as it helps to emit a loving, harmonious feeling to those you are close to. It reminds you that you are good enough and lovable.

Rose Quartz releases feelings of sadness and anger to help promote compassion, joy and peace. I had a booth at a craft fair when a woman strode up to me and demanded what exactly these stones were for. Since I was very new to this at the time, I was rather intimidated by her presence and just wished she would have walked away. But instead I asked her what was going on in her life and she told me that she was very angry because her partner had left her. I picked out a lovely Rose Quartz and gave it to her telling her to go home and hold it. She looked rather confused that I would just give her something (again, I just wanted her to go away!), and asked what the Rose Quartz was going to do for her. I said that I didn't really know but it seemed like the right stone. She walked away and I let out a sigh of relief.

A week later the woman called me on the phone and said that she was feeling much better. She took the stone home, held onto it and began crying. She cried for three days until the sadness and anger left her. Then, she said she realized that she had not wanted to be in that relationship anyway but she just didn't like how it ended. She subsequently became a good customer and believer in the energy of stones!

Fifth Chakra

Vishuddha – Purity
Color – Blue
Element – Ether or Space
Sense – Hearing
Physical Location - Throat

The fifth chakra is located in the throat and governs higher communication, speaking, hearing and listening. It helps us to understand our inner truth and convey it with our voice to the outside world.

This chakra is the center of choice and consequence, of our spiritual karma. Every choice that we make, every thought and feeling is an act of power that has biological, environmental, social, personal and global consequences.

The throat chakra is also associated with listening to one's intuition, which guides you to see your goals manifest into reality. Abundance is associated with this chakra – in the context that unconditional receiving is necessary to accept the abundance of the Universe.

It is here that we face the challenge of surrendering our own will and spirit to Divine Will. From a spiritual perspective, our highest goal is to fully release our personal will into 'the hands of the Divine' and to have faith and trust in the outcome. Many seek intuitive guidance, yet fear what that voice will have to say.

Our throat and heart chakras work together. It is difficult to be creative if you are unable to communicate your inner vision.

This charka is physically linked to our thyroid, parathyroid, jaw, neck, mouth, throat, tongue and our larynx.

Physical Imbalance: Neck and shoulder problems, jaw disorders, throat problems, underactive or overactive thyroid, hearing problems.

Emotional Imbalance: Addictions, inability to tell the truth, overly talkative or overly silent, a lack of creativity, inability to manifest or fulfill one's goals, inability to listen.

Balanced Energy: Ability to communicate, ability to create, honesty, ability to manifest, appropriate expression of feelings, humility, a connection between the heart and mind, personal integrity.

How to rebalance our heart chakra: Chanting, reading aloud, practice surrendering to the spiritual will, using your creativity, meditation, awareness of the truth.

Mantra: I am open, clear and honest.

Crystals/Stones:

Aquamarine: I call Aquamarine the "Courage to Speak" stone because it clears the throat to tell the truth of who you are and what you want. It allows for clarity of thought in order to be able to say what it is you need to say. It helps to alleviate fear so that we can move forward with clarity and self-assurance.

In 1993, I knew that I had to leave my twenty-year relationship because I was not able to become my true self in that space. I was having difficulty telling my partner that I needed to leave so I started wearing an Aquamarine pendant. I didn't automatically begin to speak but the Aquamarine made me feel so uncomfortable about not talking that I simply had to get it out.

One thing about stones, they don't automatically do your work for you – they allow you to go inside and find your answers. In this way, you are taking responsibility for your own well-being and healing. I, personally, think this is brilliant!

Aquamarine helps us to 'see' the deep part of our psyche, to explore the depths of our souls and to be honest about what we see. Courage – the courage to be you!

Blue Kyanite: Blue Kyanite is a striated stone that assists in the communication between ourself and Spirit for clear channeling of information. Its fast-acting energy works to align all of our chakras with our throat chakra.

Blue Kyanite helps with communication, clearing the throat and making speech an easier process. It is also said to be good for memory, clearing headaches and eye maladies. I also use Blue Kyanite to open sinuses. Simply place Blue Kyanite vertically directly on the sinuses and lie quietly until the sinuses open.

Blue Lace Agate: Blue Lace Agate is very useful to temper the temper. Its cool, smooth demeanor gives us pause when speaking so that there is more thoughtfulness and less spewing. It is said to be the stone of the diplomat because it helps you to develop tactfulness when speaking.

I had a client who was full of fire and just said whatever was on her mind without thinking about the effect her words were having on others. I suggested she carry Blue Lace Agate with her at all times to see if things would change. After a couple of weeks, she came into Free Spirit Crystals and asked if we had any larger pieces of the stone because she wanted to make sure she always had a sufficient amount. She said that her partner noticed almost immediately that she was speaking with more kindness and was less demanding. She wanted to make sure she always carried a blue lace agate with her!

Blue Lace Agate promotes peace and gentleness, and calms the agitation inside. It also helps with concentration and analytical thinking. Physically, it helps with ulcers and digestion.

Chrysocolla: After I was given my directive to start my crystal business, I was doing a meditation and was told that I needed to speak in front of groups to teach people about stones and healing. I immediately gave my stock answer, "No!"

Of course, I'm sure you know that the powers that be didn't give up! They said I should get some Chrysocolla and to practice talking. I had no idea what Chrysocolla was but, in that instant, I saw it with my eyes closed, written out on my forehead so I knew they meant business! So, I found a place to buy Chrysocolla and stuffed my pockets full of it. After that, I started doing classes and giving workshops on crystals and I've been doing it ever since!

This stone empowers you to let go of your self-doubt and negative beliefs about your abilities to help you bring forward your knowledge and talents. This is a great stone for teachers, orators, writers and anyone else who has a compunction to communicate with others. It helps to ground your voice and make certain that you are heard.

Chrysocolla helps with anxiety and depression, and also works with the adrenal glands and helps regulate the thyroid gland. Because it is a soft stone, it also helps to draw out inflammation so it is good for maladies of the throat chakra.

Sodalite: Sodalite helps to still the mind to allow for rational thought and speech. A great stone for public speakers, actors and singers. Sodalite helps us to gain confidence in our abilities, grounding our speech and thought so that we are centered when we need to express ourselves.

Many years ago, a customer brought her sixteen-year-old son into the store and he immediately picked up an eight-inch Sodalite wand which he began to sing into. I asked his mom why he was doing that and she replied that his dream was to be on Broadway. How interesting that he instinctively knew what stone he needed. Needless to say, she bought him the Sodalite.

A couple of years ago she came back into the store and I asked her how her son was doing. She replied that he, indeed, had gotten to Broadway and was appearing in a musical. His determination and inner desire took him exactly where he wanted to go.

Sodalite gives us a clear vision of what we want, the discipline to work for it, helps us to develop our talents and gives us the inner strength and belief in ourselves to go for it!

Turquoise: Turquoise connects our throat to both Father Sky and Mother Earth to provide balance and courage. This stone promotes leadership and authenticity allowing us to be who we are in the midst of chaos. It keeps us centered and aligned with Universal Law in order to do what it is we need to do in this life.

Turquoise is also a soft stone that helps with the respiratory system, sore throats, allergies and lung disorders. It is anti-inflammatory so it can help reduce swelling and assist in restructuring the cellular memory. Turquoise is also wonderful to use on the throat to dispel negative energies and bring in a more harmonious vibration..

Sixth Chakra

Ajna – Beyond Wisdom
Color – Indigo
Element – Knowing
Sense – Sight
Physical Location – Between Eyebrows

The third eye chakra is not only the seat of wisdom, but also a seat of conscience. This is where you not only see what is going on, but you also know what it means. This is where your sense of justice and your ethics originate. When your third eye is open, you not only see but you also understand.

This chakra is the center of our intuitive knowing; where visualization and imagination provide a springboard for inspiration. It is here that we can open ourselves to receive guidance and work with our Higher Self. And, it is through our sixth chakra that we experience telepathy, astral travel and the rediscovery of our past lives.

This chakra is physically linked to our pituitary gland, face, eyes, ears, nose, sinuses and cerebellum.

Physical Imbalance: Poor memory, eye problems, sinusitis, hearing problems, headaches, brain tumor or hemorrhage, stroke, blindness, spinal problems, learning difficulties, seizures, nightmares, hallucinations.

Emotional Imbalances: Confusion, blocked intuition, lack of inspiration, difficulty concentrating, following the crowd, inability to see the bigger picture, lack of individualism.

Balanced Energy: Purification of negative tendencies, elimination of selfish attitudes, open to receive guidance/channeling, open to telepathy, astral travel and past lives, rational thinking, power to create one's dreams, creative visualization, inspiration, developed sense of self and style, wisdom.

How to rebalance our third eye chakra: Meditation, memory exercises, alternate nostril breathing, keep a dream journal, automatic writing, relax your eye muscles, draw or do another art form that requires close observation and concentration.

Mantra: I am in touch with my deepest wisdom.

<u>Crystals/Stones:</u>

Amethyst: Amethyst is known as the "Alcoholic's Stone" because the word itself means 'not intoxicated.' It is a wonderful stone for overcoming addictions of all kinds as it helps us to understand why we developed the craving that we have in order to let go of the addiction. Healing is always about awareness, and knowing the genesis of our habits allows us the wherewithal to release them.

Not only does Amethyst allow us to break free of old habits, but it's also wonderful for letting go of old ways of thinking and believing. It helps us to move forward with a clean record, so to speak, in order to become more authentic.

Amethyst gradually opens the third eye to our own inner knowing. It assists us to develop the "Clairs" – clairvoyance, clairsentience, clairaudience. These skills can be honed through meditating with Amethyst and allowing the channels to open naturally. You can either hold an Amethyst point in your hand or place a cluster above your crown chakra when you are laying down.

Amethyst is also a wonderful mineral to use to let go of the earth plane when you are transitioning. I gave my grandmother a cluster when she was leaving us and then, when she passed, I took the Amethyst back so that I could let go of needing her to be here.

Amethyst is very calming and serene, making it a valuable tool to use when you can't sleep. Place one on your night stand or head of your bed to insure a peaceful night.

Azurite: Azurite is one of the premier stones for developing psychic ability. Its deep blue opens the chakra and connects it to the "Intergalactical Information Highway." To practice, I recommend having a specific topic for your meditation. Concentrate on uploading that topic to the Universe, then lie quietly and listen for any information that might be forth coming.

I love Azurite for its ability to unlock cellular memory and use it anywhere on the body that has a blockage or a pain. I had a client who had a pain in her hip for over a year, but had stopped going to medical doctors because they didn't know what to do for her. I placed a sizeable piece of Azurite on her hip and asked her to tell me about her injury.

She had been practicing with her softball team and had been 'tagged' by the second baseman, injuring her hip. She was angry at the manager for not telling the team to not to play so hard as it was only a practice.

After a few minutes, she mentioned that she'd been in a relationship with the team's manager but that the relationship had ended badly. Her anger had settled into her hip and could not be released until she became aware of the cause. Once she realized it, and allowed Azurite to help her work through it, the pain was released and never came back.

Azurite is a "Stone of Truth" that allows the truth to be revealed at the time that you are able to listen and incorporate the message into your consciousness.

Charoite: I call Charoite the "Kick in the Butt" stone because it works to challenge us to move forward in our lives. This lovely stone comes mainly from Siberia and has a demanding force that will not allow us to be idle. It gives us the stamina and fortitude to shift our beliefs, our habits, and our thinking in order to make a fresh start.

Charoite helps us to overcome exhaustion and keep moving forward. It assists with fear issues so that change becomes easier with each shift in consciousness.

I, personally, have used Charoite over the years when I have had difficult decisions to make and felt stagnant. I carry it in my pockets, meditate with it, and use it as a journaling tool. I love its honesty and direct energy so that I can't bluff myself into non-movement.

Lapis Lazuli: Lapis Lazuli was used in ancient times to cure mental illness. Our ancestors believed that Lapis Lazuli resolved mental confusion and brought back clarity of thought.

Lapis Lazuli is still considered to be a stone of clarity and high intellectual acuity. It sharpens the mind and assists with critical thinking. It also helps us to ascertain the truth of things to ensure that we speak and act with integrity. In so doing, it can help elevate us in our fields of endeavor.

Lapis Lazuli is good for menstrual cramps, inflammation and migraine headaches. Its Pyrite content make it a lovely stone for psychic protection. It helps in breaking down karmic patterns in order to move forward in life.

Sugilite: Sugilite is the "Purpose Stone." It calls us to create a life where we are living our soul's desire, and fulfilling what we came to earth to do. It's another stone that demands the highest ideals for our existence. It helps us to develop our inner wisdom so that we may live by Divine order and not an ego-based system.

It aligns unconditional love throughout our chakra system and grounds it in our root. Sugilite opens us to our inner calling and connection to the soul, helping us to feel the freedom in life.

Sugilite is a stone of optimism and dreams, but it asks us to let go of our old way of living in order to absorb and accept that life is magnificent and full of wonder. Use Sugilite for meditation when you desire change and encouragement from the Universal Source.

Seventh Chakra

Sahasrara – 1,000 Petal Lotus
Color – Violet
Element – Cosmic Energy
Sense – Thought (To Know)
Physical Location – Above Head

The crown chakra oversees the brain, the top of the head, our hormones and nervous system. When it is out of balance you may experience a sensitivity to light and a chronic tiredness.

It receives energy to sustain life and it gives back the personal energy to unite with the collective pool of consciousness. It is the meeting point between finite (your body and your ego) and infinite (the universe and your soul).

This chakra is about selflessness, humanitarianism and integrating the whole of who we are. Our crown chakra helps us understand that part of our life lesson is about experiencing the Divine and learning to understand the Divine meaning in our life.

The challenge of this chakra is to liberate the Spirit – to open to the Divine – and, at the same time, to stay firmly rooted deep in the ground. It is associated with peace, understanding and knowledge, enlightenment, conscious awareness and divinity.

This chakra is physically linked to our cerebral cortex, central nervous system and pineal gland.

Unbalanced Energy: Feeling of being disconnected spiritually, a lack of direction or purpose, a sense of being lost or incomplete, depression, confusion, loss of faith, mentally disconnected, dementia, epilepsy, schizophrenia, light sensitivity, headaches, autoimmune disorders, neurological disorders.

Balanced Energy: Serenity, joy and deep peace about life, a sense of knowing that there is a deeper meaning of life and that there is an order that underlies all of existence, a feeling of oneness with the Universe.

How to rebalance our crown chakra: Meditation, grounding, carrying crystals, spiritual awareness.

Mantra: I honor the Divine within me.

Crystals/Stones:

Fluorite: Fluorite is the best stone I know for mental assimilation, concentration and helping to clear scattered thought patterns. It assists with memory and mental clarity in order to keep the mind sharp for making decisions. It's wonderful for students who have difficulty retaining information, for people who have jobs that require mental concentration, for computer technicians and teachers.

When I was in high school, I was a straight C student, throwing in an occasional A or B for music class and English. I was not good at memorizing, and would cry when I had to memorize something to recite.

After I hurt my arm, I decided to go back to school because I couldn't really do anything else. I took classes that required me to retain large amounts of information. My friend, Patty, gave me a piece of Fluorite and I would hold it when I studied. Much to my amazement, I got straight A's in college!

Another time I went to Melody's teacher class but I had not taken her other classes so I didn't have the basic information to build on. I studied with a piece of Fluorite in hand. At night, I placed that along with a double terminated crystal on the packet of information facing my head at night. I passed the test with only seven answers wrong out of 140 questions! Needless to say, I'm a big fan of Fluorite.

Herkimer Diamond: Herkimer Diamonds are great for inspiring and remembering dreams, and assist with clairvoyance and clairaudience. Said to be the most powerful of all the quartz crystals, each Herkimer is double terminated, giving it the power to transmute negative energy and to clear the mind. It is a wonderful amplifier of energy and helps to bring in messages and information from Universe.

I had a friend who purchased several Hermiker diamonds and placed them in her pillow case so that she would have more lucid dreams. The next morning, her husband told her about all the amazing dreams he had. The energy in this stone will transfer!

Herkimer's can also assist in removing energy blocks from our minds in order to assist in transferring telepathic thoughts.

Quartz Crystal: Quartz Crystal has the closest vibration to that of the human body than any other mineral, which is why it is so effective with physical healing. It purifies, energizes, balances, and restructures energy in the body. If I could have only one type of stone, it would be Quartz Crystal.

Quartz is an electromagnetic force which energizes whatever it connects with. Our bodies are also electromagnetic. Matching quartz to the body moves energy, and brings the body back to its natural vibration.

Electronics such as cell phones, television sets, computers and watches all run with quartz energy. It is the second most ubiquitous mineral on earth next to gypsum and does more than any other stone.

Rutilated Quartz: Rutilated Quartz has metal filament inside of quartz crystal, intensifying the energy of the quartz. This allows the energy to go beneath the surface of energy blocks in order to bring up whatever issue or stuck emotion is present. It is a fast-acting stone that is useful in lifting out the blockages. It is also helpful for exhaustion and energy depletion.

This stone will intensify whatever emotion is below the surface of our psyche. I once gave my sister a sizeable chunk of Rutilated Quartz to use. She called me one day crying that her entire family was in an angry uproar, and that she believed the crystal to be evil.

My first thought was, "Aha, it's working!" I told her to wrap the crystal in a towel and to place it in the garage away from the family. And when she did, things went back to the way they were previously. But, this illustrated that this stone helped to expel the negativity that was present in my sister's home environment.

Rutilated Quartz is excellent for enhancing your telepathic abilities and for doing channeling work. I suggest you either have a scribe or record your sessions.

Selenite: I call Selenite the "Rocket Ship" because it has very fast energy that can remove blockages in our body and rapidly clear the meridians. Although it is a crown chakra stone, I use it all over the body to move energy. If someone comes in feeling sluggish and tired, I place Selenite both in between and outside the legs to facilitate movement. I will also place Selenite below the feet, at the root chakra and proceed up the chakra system. This assists the physical body to not have to work so hard to open things up. Selenite activates all our chakras.

Selenite can also clear the mind and speed up the process of telecommunication with the Universe. It assists us in developing telepathic communication skills and psychic abilities. It's a fabulous stone for channeling information.

I use Selenite after I finish a session on someone to clear the aura on all seven levels of the energy field. This leaves the client feeling like they've had an energy bath!

Chapter Six

Additional Healing Stones

The stones in this section are mainly used for opening the connections to our

spiritual guidance, although there are a few that deal with the lower chakras. As we

continue to expand our awareness and become more spiritually refined, the tools we

need will be more energetically intense, assisting us to open to and understand more

complex information and concepts. This is not to say that they are more important than

the other minerals, but opening to our guidance is a progressive process and we can't

skip steps along the way.

I encourage people to start slowly and add new stones to your educational repertoire

as you progress. Each one has its own qualities and vibrations to help you open to

yourself and spirit. Also, just as with anything else, some stones work differently for

some than for others. It is through usage and experimentation that we come up with

the combinations that will work properly for us.

Not everyone tolerates substances the same way. In the same way that some of us

are allergic to strawberries while others thrive with their nutrients, if one stone doesn't work for you as it is described, try something else. And, remember, when you use a new stone, journal what you feel, think, and experience afterwards. This will help you to keep track of what works for you, how it works, and to give you the building blocks to build on.

I obviously can't write about every single stone – there isn't enough time or energy for me to do so. But the stones we discuss in this book will give you what you need to transform your life.

<u>Amazonite</u>

Amazonite is a stone of courage and helps to heal emotional disturbances and self-defeating behaviors as it takes internal courage to face one's flaws and make the decision to change. It allows us to see our ego for what it is and not allow it to run our lives without first consulting our spirit to bring clarity to our thoughts and feelings.

Amazonite helps us to find harmony in our chaos by showing us how our fears control the truth of who we are and giving us a more worry free state of mind. This is a wonderful stone for those working on trauma issues as it helps to soothe and regulate the nervous system bringing in a more calm state of being.

Amazonite is also useful for deflecting the electromagnetic field of computers, cell phones, television sets and microwaves.

<u>Amethyst - Chevron</u>
Chevron Amethyst is a purple stone with white markings in the form of a Vee. It

combines the strengthening qualities of quartz with the stress relieving qualities of amethyst. This form of Amethyst enhances peace of mind, relaxation, courage and inner strength. As with totally purple Amethyst, it is used in breaking old patterns and addictions allowing us to let go of things that are not for our higher purpose. Chevron Amethyst helps us to connect to the truth of the Universe providing a path towards enlightenment.

Ametrine

Ametrine is a combination of Amethyst and Citrine giving it the qualities of both minerals. Amethyst is the stone of letting go and Citrine is the stone of releasing fear so they work hand in hand to help us understand why we hold onto the things we do in order to release what we no longer need. This can apply to thoughts, old beliefs, old patterns, resentments, people who no longer belong in our lives, a job that doesn't satisfy you – and the list goes on and on. It helps to release negative emotional programming and negative memories in order to transform emotional blocks and move into a more freeing state of being.

Ametrine aids in meditation, boosting our psychic abilities and helping us to believe that we are more than the sum parts of our human bodies. It helps us to understand that there is more to this world then we have been taught and that the Universe has unlimited possibilities for us. Thus, Ametrine is a wonderful asset in manifesting and shaping our lives as we would like them to be, not what we were taught they should be.

<u>Angelite</u>

Angelite is a stone of serenity, inner peace and calm. It helps to dispel fear and anger and encourages forgiveness. It enhances telepathy, psychic awareness and astral travel. It creates a shield of psychic protection while communicating with your guides and angels.

Angelite is a stone of détente bringing tact and compassion in communication. It helps you to speak your truth and inspires forgiveness in order to smooth out old contentious situations. It brings deeper understanding of the human condition to bring healing on all levels of the auric field.

Physically Angelite bolsters the throat chakra, helps to balance the thyroid, thymus and reduce inflammation. It can be useful for headaches and the circulatory system.

<u>Apatite</u>

Apatite is a wonderful stone for helping us to break addictions and old belief patterns. It helps us to focus on what is most important and expands our curiosity for knowledge and truth thereby enhancing our imagination and intuition. It helps us to develop our memory, is a useful tool for studying and stimulate thoughts and ideas.

Apatite can enable us to break out of patterns of shyness and self-consciousness in order to build self-reliance so that we can be more outgoing and social. It helps to balance the throat chakra so that we can express ourselves more freely and honestly.

Apatite can also help us develop our psychic senses whether that be clairvoyance, clairaudience or clairsentience. Please know that everyone has these abilities but sometimes they need to be honed and Apatite is a stone that can open those lines of communication.

Apophyllite

You can identify an Apophyllite crystal its flat top – it looks like a mesa. Apophyllite is a clear, soft stone that is perfect for meditation because its clarity connects to the etheric realms very quickly. It helps us to see the truth of the world and to be able to take that truth and live it inside of us. I believe it to be a stone of spiritual transformation as it helps us to self-reflect on our behavior, correct it and live in honesty.

You can use Apophyllite for scrying (staring into the crystal), for developing your psychic abilities, and for seeing into the future. If you get a pyramid shaped piece instead of a cluster, lie on a flat surface and place it on your third eye for clarity. I call this the truth teller as it will be very direct and use its energy to help shift your beliefs from fear based to love based.

Boji Stones

Mainly found in Kansas, Boji Stones are made up primarily of Pyrite and are said to be as old as the earth itself. These stones are usually sold in pairs as they are identified as male and female with the male stones having bumps and sharper edges and the female being smooth. For balance, it is helpful to have them both be the same size.

Boji stones assist in balancing the male and female energies and help to align the chakras. I like to hold the male Boji in the left hand and the female Boji in the right hand even though the left is said to be female and the right is said to embody male energy. I find that this helps give each side the opposite energy in order to balance it. Boji stones help to clear chakras, help to heal emotional issues, and is used to promote regeneration of damaged cellular tissue.

When I see a client who either has too much aggression or is too meek, I have them hold the Boji stones to assist with balancing the polarities of the body. I have them place the stones in the palms of the hands to allow the energy to flow throughout the nervous system. I also find that doing this helps to bring calm and peace.

<u>Calcites</u>

There over 800 different Calcites available to us but I will concentrate on three of them otherwise this whole book would be Calcite driven! There is a Calcite for each chakra so you could do an entire chakra bath using this stone. I have actually done that and it is very soothing and made me want to sleep. Just collect the corresponding colored Calcite for each chakra and allow yourself a luxurious half hour of peace!

Calcite has a 3 hardness on the Mohs scale so it acts as a drawing out agent for the body thus cleansing the cells of old stuck memories and giving release to the tension that these memories cause. Calcite is very calming and assists in leveling out our moods in order to find peace.

Blue Calcite

Blue Calcite is used in the area of communication and thoughts. It helps us to release rigidity in order to see the bigger picture and allows us to foster positive communication with those who may have a different viewpoint, softening argumentation. It aids in being able to express our beliefs and opinions calmly and without anger.

Physically, Blue Calcite is appropriate for high blood pressure, releasing tension in the joints, soothing lung and throat maladies and regulating the thyroid.

Green Calcite

Green Calcite is wonderful for what I call the "itises" – arthritis, bursitis, tendonitis - which means inflammation. Because it is a soft stone, it helps to draw out the heat and inflammation caused by these afflictions. Simply place the Calcite directly on the pain for as long as necessary and you should find relief.

Green Calcite also releases limiting beliefs brought on by fear and releases rigid thinking. It calms angry energy (which is inflammation) and allows one to go through transitions more gracefully.

Orange Calcite

Orange Calcite is useful on the second chakra to gently draw out blockages which prevent us from knowing our passion in life. It creates a safe place inside where we can explore our creative nature and understand how we might manifest our dreams. Unlike the Ruby which will demand and push, Orange Calcite takes its time to assist in bringing out the confidence to know our gifts proceed on an inventive level.

Calcite Rhomboids

A rhomboid has six parallel planes (visualize this as top, bottom, side, side, end, end) all connected to each other. Its points help with connection and interconnection with parallel planes of reality. It assists in connecting to the God source to show us that God is not "out there" but inside of us allowing us to realize our own divinity.

The Calcite Rhomboid helps us to understand and release the negative behavioral patterns that prevent us from knowing that we are God – that our connectedness to the God-Source is because we are a part of the spark that created all that is. This important knowledge allows us to know our magnificence and live in harmony with all creation.

To use a Calcite Rhomboid, lay on a flat surface and place the stone above your head with the thinner angles facing the head and pointing towards the 12th chakra. If you want to add to the intensity of the layout, place Rhomboids beneath your feet with the same configuration to allow the energy to reach from your root to the outer chakras and beyond.

Celestite

This heavenly blue stone is one of the best for connecting to Spirit and the angelic realm. Its soft nature peacefully brings us into meditation with our guides and raises our consciousness to a new spiritual level. It helps us to alleviate our fear and worry while at the same time purifying our aura and chakras.

Celestite assists with clearing mental disorders by helping us to "see" a different way to live in this world. It changes our paradigm of what is real and what is not by expanding our perceptions. It gives us the purview to live beyond the mundane and know that what we experience here on earth is for lesson learning and growing spiritually.

Celestite helps to clear negative energy out of one's environment and bring in a calm serenity. It assists in dispelling fear, anxiety, worry and depression by lifting the shroud of disillusionment about life. It aids in expanding one's imagination in order to create a sane world in which they can live peacefully.

Chalcedony

Chalcedony is a stone that helps to promote joy by reducing negativity in one's field. It shows where we hold that negativity inside, why we feel the need to be negative and brings us an emotional honesty in order to filter out the glass is half empty mentality.

Chalcedony assists with nurturing calm, peace and good will for all by bringing in feelings of benevolence and altruism. It transforms sadness into joy, hostility into peace and discord into harmony.

This stone is also helpful in connecting to spirit guides and angels in order to understand our own need to shift and change into more loving, forgiving beings.

<u>Chiastolite</u>

Chiastolite is a brown stone that can be identified by the graphite cross that runs through each slice, thus its name – the Cross Stone.

Chiastolite is helpful for bringing balance and harmony, stability and grounding. You can either hold it or place it on the second chakra although I don't have any concrete rules about where to place the stones. It assists with problem solving and memory as it helps in balancing the male/female sides of the brain to bring practical thinking. It aids in awakening spiritual awareness and making it a practical part of one's life. It is also useful for blood disorders, veins, blood circulation and easing blood pressure.

Chiastolite is also good for protecting the energy field from negative influences giving a feeling of security and help in feeling calm in the midst of turmoil. It is a good stone to use when you are feeling unstable and need a more practical outlook.

<u>Chlorite</u>

Chlorite is a soft green mineral often found inside of quartz crystals. It looks moss-like and allows the crystal to amplify the energy of the Chlorite.

Chlorite is one of the most powerful healing stones. It cleanses and purifies the aura and chakras and removes negative energy of all kinds including anger and hostility. It is a wonderful stone for cleansing the blood and working with the respiratory system. Holding it in your hands, placing it on the lungs, liver, spleen, intestines, stomach and adrenal glands is a great way to allow the vibration to circulate through the body.

Chlorite helps us to understand compassion and how we, individually, can connect to that part of ourselves by finding self-compassion in order to have compassion for all. This mineral has a softness, a sweetness that allows us to feel our feelings so that we may heal from the effects of those which we have stifled throughout the years. Gentility is the modus operandi of Chlorite as we allow it to patiently work on those parts of us that need its tender healing care.

Copper

Copper is probably the best conductor of electricity for the body. All of our nerve endings are in the palms of our hands and bottoms of our feet so when we hold copper in our hands, the energy travels through our nervous system to balance it. This is perfect for everyone as the nervous system is the "brain" of our physical body. All parts of our body are run by the nervous system – if it breaks down, we break down. Holding copper everyday helps to keep things running more smoothly.

Copper connects with the energies from higher planes and helps with increasing our energy levels. It also helps with the synapses of the brain, circulation in the body and supports red blood cells and tissues. Copper is also useful for alleviating the pain of arthritis. Many people wear copper bracelets for pain reduction and nerve rejuvenation.

Great conductor of energy from electricity to subtle energies from higher planes; enhances the transmission of thoughts and long distance healing; arthritis, low energy, relieves pain of broken bones, sprains and strains. Balancing and helps with low energy levels.

Coral

Coral is the lungs of the sea and represents a flow of energy that lives in harmony with all living organisms in its environment. It allows us to understand how we, also, need to do the same in our own worlds. It helps to connect with nature, attracts love and prosperity, assists us with knowing our passionate nature, gives us a more optimistic outlook and shows us our creative side. Using Coral gives us a sense of inner peace, inner strength and understanding of purpose.

Physically, it assists with the blood and circulatory systems, kidneys, bladder, bones and bone marrow and the respiratory system.

Danburite

Danburite is either pink or clear and has striations on its main body. The tip comes to a flat shape with a straight tip making it very recognizable from other stones. Oftentimes you will see rainbows inside.

Danburite is a stone of joy and open-heartedness. It connects the crown chakra to the heart, opening blockages which prevent us from finding happiness. It brings clarity in issues of pride and ego, giving us an indication of how we allow said ego to run rampant in our lives and distort our joy. Danburite's mission is to help us find the bliss of our existence by letting go of useless hurts, grudges and misunderstandings. It seeks cooperation, not competition and gives us a freedom from emotional pain by showing us how to forgive and forget.

<u>Emeralds</u>

This lovely gem stone is the seeker of the truth, going to places inside of your heart where you hide from yourself or deceive yourself. It allows us to let go of the secrets of the past in order to find a new beginning and refresh the joy in our lives.

Emeralds also help with mental clarity and intuition, bringing in knowledge of the heart of the Universe to allow us to open our minds and bring in the wisdom to perceive and understand Love. It allows us to visualize that which we desire and know that all things are possible.

It is said to be the stone of romance and faithfulness which also includes being faithful to our own selves and our own journeys. It is also useful for lifting depression and strengthening memory.

<u>Galena</u>

Galena is the primary source of lead and is a very heavy stone but, in spite of its weight, it is only a 2.5 hardness on the Mohs scale making it very soft. As we know from the guidelines for using stones, soft stones draw out inflammation and blocked energy. Galena also helps with increasing the circulation in the body. It is good for joint pain and to stimulate the nervous system.

As we know, a lead vest is used when we get x-rays to absorb radiation and I know x-ray technicians who carry Galena in their pockets just as a preventative measure.

My favorite use for Galena is its ability to absorb radiation from all of the electronics that we now have in our homes. I have a large piece in front of my television set and use it near my microwave. It's helpful to have Galena at your computer station and when using any Wi-Fi device and to place it around electrical outlets.

<u>Garnet</u>

Garnets have been used as far back as the Bronze Age in central Europe and 5,000 years ago in Egypt. It was mentioned as one of the gem stones used in breast plates of seers and the High Priest and Priestesses. It is a stone of truth and faith and is believed to be a cleansing and purifying agent.

Garnets enhance romantic love, passion, sensuality, sexuality and intimacy. They promote positive thinking and self-confidence allowing one to develop their creativity and passions. It is said to enhance one's career by developing the ability to manifest.

This is a stone of health helping to dissolve negative energy by cleansing and purifying the systems of the body. It's good for circulatory system and is useful with depression and anxiety.

Garnets help us to understand our worth and how we can overcome our past in order to be of service to the present. They represent courage and fortitude to move forward.

<u>Hiddenite</u>

Hiddenite is a cousin of Kunzite and is a hard, green striated mineral allowing for a lovely flow of energy from one chakra to another. While Kunzite is the "Love Stone of the 21st Century" for its ability to help us love ourselves, Hiddenite also assists in going deep into the heart to find the truth of one's relationship to self. Sometimes I will use both of them together to combine the pink and green vibrations in order to maximize the energy of both colors.

Hiddenite helps to support the emotions enabling us to stay steady and not go into an abyss of unorganized feelings. It also supports us in times of loss and grief, showing us that we are capable of reaching down deep and finding the self-love and soothing that we need. In that vein, it helps engender compassion for ourselves and encompasses the bond of trust to relationships.

Hiddenite is said to attract abundance by illustrating to us our own abilities to see our worth and goodness.

Howlite

Howlite is a white stone that is connected with spiritual guidance and purity.

The black streaks that run through it help to connect the crown chakra to the root in order to bring that guidance and purity down through the entire body.

Howlite helps to dispel a critical state of mind and judgmentalism bringing peace and calm to one's being. It helps to dispel the effects of selfishness, rudeness, and the pain of stress. It teaches us that love is all there is – everything else is fear and fear brings pain and discomfort.

Placing a sizeable piece of Howlite in your environment will bring calm and ease as it works on removing anger and hostility in your aura. It aids in helping you to understand why you have anger or rage and to see the underlying sadness that has resulted in that anger.

This mineral is also said to assist with strengthening bones, teeth, calcium levels and alleviate leg cramps.

<u>Hypersthene</u>

Hypersthene is a gray/black mineral with beautiful chatoyancy who's name is derived from the Greek meaning "extreme strength". It assists in enhancing self-esteem and helps to put one at ease in social situations by helping to alleviate shyness. Before it can do that, however, it will bring to awareness the issues one has about personal issues revolving around feelings of self-worth. Hypersthene is a stone of courage giving one the fortitude to examine and shift how they feel about themselves in order to bring self-respect and non-judgmentalism to one's life.

Hypersthene is also a stone of problem solving, boosting energy to being self-reliant and self-sufficient in standing up on one's own two feet and knowing that we have all of our own answers inside.

Hypersthene is also a fine tool for assisting with enhancing clairaudience and psychic abilities. It connects to the etheric realm while at the same time bringing grounding energy down from the crown chakra. This insures that we remain centered on the earth while connecting to spirit.

<u>Jade</u>

Jade is a stone for abundance and bountiful gardens and harvests. If you relate that to the bounty that you have inside of yourself, use Jade to harvest your ideas, your creativity and your fortitude to achieve what you wish to achieve. Jade is a stone for wisdom and emotional stability allowing us to use all of our talents and knowledge for the good of all.

Jade is a sweet stone that helps us to bring in the love that we desire but showing us the love that is inside of us. It brings balance to our lives by showing us that love can solve all issues and to not let our minds and egos inflate the stories we are being told or that we imagine. It stabilizes the personality and brings harmony while attracting good luck and friendship.

Jade is also known as the "Dream Stone" for its ability to help us create and remember our dreams. Some people like to place it on their third eye when they fall asleep in order to have a faster connection to the other dimensions and bring insightful dreams and emotional release.

Physically, Jade is useful for cleansing toxins from the body, balancing bodily fluids and diminishing cramping.

K-2

The K-2 stone comes from the mountains of Pakistan and is a relatively new find. It is a combination of Granite and Azurite giving it both a grounding effect and a spiritual connection. The beauty of this stone is that it helps you stay connected to the earth while allowing you to explore celestial regions of the Universe. When used in meditation, it can give you peace of mind that you will be safe and secure while you find your spiritual home.

K-2 also assists in opening your 6th chakra or 3rd eye to more psychic sensing and making the process practical. Yes, there is practical psychic exploration!!

Labradorite

In Inuit lore, Labradorite fell out of the sky from the Aurora Borealis bringing with it the vibrant colors and chatoyancy of its surging colors. Labradorite is known as the "Stone of Magic" as its mysteries help us to unlock the spiritual magic inside of ourselves. It is a stone of transformation bringing clarity and insight into our destinies. It aids in increasing our intuition and psychic ability as well as bring us clear dreams for our futures.

It is a stone of actualization, grounding the spiritual into each of our chakras and allowing us to sit with the knowing that we are far more then we realize. Labradorite gives us a sense of what lies before us as we seek the ultimate bliss of our existence and guides us through that adventure with curiosity and fascination.

Labradorite is the finest stone I know for repelling negative energies and influences around you whether that be in your home, work environment or gloomy pessimistic people in your life. Wear a piece as jewelry, keep some in your pocket, place it on your desk at work or in several places at home to rebuff those energies.

Stone of transformation; clear, balance and protect the aura; clarity and insight into our destinies; attracts success; dream recall and using dreams in everyday life; stress and anxiety reduction; increases intuition and psychic ability; helps realize and achieve your destiny while enhancing faith and reliance in yourself.

Lingam

Lingams are oval shaped stones from India which are formed by rolling in the Narmada river until they are smooth and are collected from the river in the dry season. They are the sacred stone of the Hindu religion and are used in ceremonies. When I was studying with Katrina Raphaell in Hawaii, we went to a temple where they had a Lingam several feet tall and did a ritual using rose petals.

The shape of the Lingam represents the male energy while the markings represent the female energy giving it a unifying force. Lingams help to balance the energy field and assist in generating one's creativity giving birth to one's ideas. Some say they are useful for infertility and reproduction. They instill a sacred attitude in all aspects of life and assist with the rising of the Kundalini.

I like to place a Lingam sideways in between the ankles with a quartz crystal point on each side pointing towards the ankle. It is very grounding and helps the client to remain anchored during a session. I will also have the client hold a smaller Lingam in each hand to help with stability. This is very helpful if the client is ungrounded, anxious or unfocused.

Moldavite

Moldavite is an olive to forest green colored specimen formed by a meteor impact in Europe about 15 million years ago. This wrinkly looking pieces are one of the only space "stones" that we have and can be considered an extraterrestrial gemstone.

The first time someone put Moldavite into my palm, I dropped it immediately as I was not ready for the impact it would have on my life. The energy was very strong and felt demanding to me, something that I was not prepared for at the time. It was a few years after that when I became acquainted with it again that I was able to use it as I had done much more work on myself and was no longer afraid to move forward.

Moldavite is cosmically expansive and is known as the stone of transformation. It raises the vibration of everything around it and brings up issues that need to be revamped and reconstructed. It strengthens your cosmic connection and consciousness while expanding your belief in what is cosmically possible. It allows for communication with interdimensional forces and gives us insight into the far reaches of the Universe.

This is a mineral for the mystic, the seer, the seeker, the one who wishes to go beyond what is seen with the earthly eye.

<u>Morganite</u>

Morganite is a pink cousin of Aquamarine in the Beryl family and, like Aquamarine, is a stone of honesty and truth. Used on the heart, this stone will bring up the truth so that there is no fooling one's self about their life and what they need to resolve in order to live a totally honest life with themselves. At the same time, it emphasizes using compassion, patience and empathy in order to temper what may arise.

Morganite brings in and rekindles love, both for the self and for others on a Divine level. It aids in forgiveness and balances the emotions. It helps to release old trauma and past issues to clear space for new and exciting love to enter with confidence.

Morganite is the stone of fairness, giving one tact and reason to any situation. It helps to balance both sides of a question in order to find the most equitable solution. This is a wonderful stone for openness and communication in relationships keeping both sides aware of all possibilities and assists in seeing the fears that stifle moving forward.

Morganite also aids in seeing the big picture of our spiritual connections, of our soul's desires and who we truly are in the scheme of the Universe. Work with this when you want to break free of small concepts of who you are and to understand your magnificence in the scope of ALL.

Nuummite

Nuummite is a hard black stone with silver and gold specks that was first discovered in Greenland in 1982 making it a relatively "young" stone in healing terms although it started forming in the earth three billion years ago. The hardness of Nuumite makes it an effective tool for going into deep blockages in the body to retrieve locked memories and past life issues.

Nuummite brings protection from negative forces and integrates pieces which have been separated from the self. It's useful for soul retrieval work and mental and psychic healing.

I like placing Nuummite on a client's body when I work in the layers of the auric field as it helps to repair tears and holes in the aura. It emits a protective layer of energy to prevent outside forces from entering in when doing this vulnerable work. I also recommend carrying Nuummite if you're feeling very sensitive and exposed as it helps with feeling safe.

Pietersite

Pietersite is one of the most beautiful stones I know of and one of my favorites. I've been carrying Pietersite with me for years and feel naked without it. It gives me a sense of who I am in this world and helps me stay steady within myself as I face various situations in life. It was named after Syd Pieters from South Africa where he discovered it.

Pietersite, according to Melody, is said to contain the kingdom of heaven, dispelling illusions and assisting in the recognition of the beauty of the soul. It cuts through the fog of this world and helps us to see the truth of the Universe in order to not get caught in the tangled web of lies that we have been taught since we were created. It shows us the Light of the Universe, where we came from, what our destinies are and how we can move through to realize who we truly are. As Melody says, "That's quite a stone, Syd!"

Petrified Wood

Petrified Wood is formed when silicon oxide enters a tree and crystalizes the wood. The rings of the tree represent the ages and growth of our lives analogously showing us how we grow from the inside out. It sets an example of how we can grow our roots to steady our lives and become internally strong and healthy.

Petrified Wood assists in grounding in order to calm fears and stabilize emotions based on survival. It aids in building strong bones, alleviating backaches, conditioning the skin and rejuvenating the hair. The common denominator in all of these things is taking care of our inner selves so that the outer self is healthy. Petrified Wood reminds us that our core will determine how we present ourselves to the world.

I like to use Petrified Wood for past life remembrance and breaking karmic patterns as it connects to the roots of beginnings and allows us to understand the patterns that we need to heal in order to become our true selves. I'll place it at the feet, in the middle of the legs and on the second chakra to allow the energy to percolate throughout the root area. Bringing up awareness of these patterns assist us in letting go of what is no longer useful for our growth. It can also aid in pointing out our talents and gifts so that we can grow these as well.

<u>Shungite</u>

Over two billion years old, Shungite is one of the most useful stones to appear on the healing scene. It is one of the only known natural material known to contain fullerenes, which are powerful anti-oxidants. Fullerenes are said to absorb and eliminate anything that is a health hazard to human life. Shungite is used to filter water and infuse it with healing properties for the body.

This soft, black mineral is a staple for anyone that owns electronic devices as it repels the electromagnetic field from those devices away from you. Place it in your pockets, your billfold, near your television sets, your microwave, your computers, and hand held devices. We have Shungite that you can place on the back of your cell phones to negate the EMFs coming toward you.

This is another stone that I carry with me constantly to ward off all of the unwanted electromagnetic energy coming at us every day.

Spirit Quartz

Spirit Quartz is lavender-colored drusy Amethyst cluster with a plethora of tiny crystals on the same base. Each one of these crystal points emits white light into the environment helping to clear negativity and bring a sense of calm and peace to the area.

Spirit Quartz also brings cohesiveness to a group showing us that by honoring the divinity in one another, we can work and live together with mutual cooperation and respect.

This stone also helps us move through transitions in our lives with understanding and grace, providing the self-compassion we need to express our emotions and release the past. It will cleanse and balance the chakras and fill any voids with positive energy.

Super Seven

The Super Seven is so named because it contains seven different minerals: Amethyst, Clear Quartz, Smoky Quartz, Cacoxenite, Rutile, Goethite and Lepidocrocite. This stone takes on the qualities of all seven minerals and is said to be the stone of higher consciousness. It helps to align and balance our chakras with the

Divine giving whoever uses it the awareness of true healing for the world. It is a stone that must be used responsibly for the betterment of all – it is not an element that is used primarily for the self. Whoever is attracted to the Super 7 has an innate knowledge of what must be done to heal the whole world, not just themselves. Melody says it brings the soul back into communication with the Divine. It stimulates all aspects of psychic development but must be used consciously and ethically.

Sleeping with a Super 7 helps you to shift spiritually and bring you closer to the secrets of the Universe.

<u>Tourmalines</u>

Just as with Calcites, there are many different colors of Tourmaline, enough to do an entire chakra balancing. The striated nature of Tourmaline gives it a speedy energy that helps to open and balance chakras with ease. Depending upon the color, each one works on a specific chakra to help clear away negative emotional patterns and release past cellular memory. Once that is accomplished, the Tourmaline helps to purify and renew the cellular structure and enliven the parts of you that have been cleared.

Tourmaline assists in diffusing and alleviating negative energies giving you a sense of calm and clarity. Because it is quite hard and striated, it helps you get right to the issue to clear up confusion, obstructed thought patterns and issues from the past. It is a very protective stone so it will shield your psyche when doing deep process work.

Tourmalines transmute negative energy into positive energy making them very useful for those of us who tend to be glass half full types. It gives us a sense of the goodness in the world as it helps us to see the goodness in our own selves.

Unakite

Unakite is a double heart stone as it is both pink and green in color. It assists us in letting go of self-judgment in order to feel unconditional love for ourselves and others. It is a wonderful stone to use for healing emotional issues and releasing pain from the past so that we can move forward in a more positive, loving way.

Unakite is a lovely stone to use for healing abandonment and separation issues (which, in my very humble opinion, we all have on some level). It gives us a sense of our internal strength in order to be self-sufficient and self-reliant while at the same time being vulnerable enough to ask for help when we need it.

This gentle yet powerful mineral also aids in pregnancy and childbirth, giving the mother a more moderate pregnancy with awareness of her own process.

Unakite also is a great stone for connecting with one's animal guides.

Healing Techniques

Chapter Seven

Conducting a Healing Session

Once you know the guidelines for stone/crystal healing, you can do a layout using the KISS Guide to Layouts. As with any energy healing modality, these are simply guidelines. There are many other models, so I encourage you to use your own discretion and experience when doing healing work.

It is important to have a comfortable, safe environment for your client. Make sure that your room is private, at a comfortable temperature, with the lights dimmed. Have pillows, blankets and knee bolsters available for their comfort.

Prior to the client's arrival, cleanse the room by smudging or using the laser wand technique. For this technique, clear the laser wand, point the crystal toward the wall and walk around the room creating a protective barrier. You may want to say a blessing as you walk around the room.

Next, discuss with your client the reason for his/her visit, and how they would like you to proceed with the session. Ask if they want a blanket, a pillow, and if they would like soft music playing in the background.

Place your hands on their feet to gain a sense of what is happening energetically in their body, aura, and emotional system. All of the nerve endings of the body are in the palms of the hands and bottoms of the feet so that, when you connect to their feet, you are connecting to their nervous system.

This is a wonderful connection for identifying the energy flow in their body. Here is where you will begin to ascertain which stones to use for the session. Continue to work up the legs, torso and arms with your hands, gently feeling in to access information on how to proceed with the healing. Their body will tell you what stones are needed. Trust your feelings and instincts! I always tell my students to take their heads off and use all of their senses to determine which stones to use.

Choose the stones and clear them before you place them on the body. As a reminder, always clear the stones before and after a session. Stones can pick up the energy of the person being worked on, so it is imperative to clear the stones each time you use them.

If you are unsure of what stones to place on your client, use the basic chakra layout in Chapter 2. You can also refer to the KISS Guide to Stone Layouts book for a specific layout for your client.

Beginning at the feet, place the stones where you FEEL they need to be. This helps to keep your client as grounded as possible during their session. Work your way up the body from the root chakra to the crown.

Do whatever energy work in which you are well-versed. If you have not learned how to do energy work, simply allow your client to lie on the table with the layout. The stones will do what they are meant to do for each individual. If, during the session, a certain stone does not feel right to your client, remove it.

When finished, remove the stones starting from the head and working your way down to their feet. Again, we want our clients to be as grounded as possible. Removing the grounding stones first may cause your client to lose their center.

Take a moment to clear the stones, then clear the client's aura either by doing an aura sweep or by lightly raking their arms and legs with your fingertips. Never touch anyone inappropriately during a session!

Check to make sure your client is grounded and centered after their session. Look into their eyes and verify that they don't have a dreamy, far-away look. Rub their back, rub their feet, or crawl your fingers alongside their spine from the bottom up. A wonderful way to get them back to full awareness is to have them hold a sizeable piece of hematite in each hand. Remember, you are responsible for your client being present and accounted for. Do not let them drive if they are not fully in their body!

Note: If you want to also work in the levels of the field, please make sure that you practice, practice, practice!!

Chapter Eight

Levels of the Auric Field

When learning how to do energy work, it is necessary to work not just on the physical body, but the levels of energy patterns that surround the body as well. These are known as levels or layers of the field and are separate from the seven chakras. There are seven levels above the physical body, each one having their own characteristics, and hold information about our current life, our past lives, our health, our beliefs and our wounds. These levels cover the entire body both front and back and the events of our lives exist energetically in the layers of the field. Developing your subtle sense perception will assist you in "feeling" into the layers so that you can do energy work in the auric field.

There may be blockages in the levels which may feel different to each person. Some of them may feel like a tar-like substance, prickly, hot or cold. Some layers might feel like there are holes or spongy or buoyant. There may be spots that feel like there are knots or places that feel oily and slick. Again, everyone will experience them differently because each person has their own way of feeling energy.

Every healing practitioner that I know has developed their own way of feeling and sensing this – there is no one right way. The most important thing to remember when working in the levels of the field is to keep your head and your ego out of it. If you find yourself thinking about what you are feeling, then you are not feeling – you are thinking. And, while we do need to be educated with the knowledge of each practice, it is when you allow your senses to become the teacher that you can ultimately sense things without judgment. That is why I urge everyone to practice, practice, practice feeling into the levels of the field before beginning to use crystals and stones to work on the blockages.

Healing is feeling and feeling is healing. One of my students taught me this – she tapped her head and repeated stupid, stupid, stupid, and then rubbed her hand and repeated smart, smart, smart. Our ego mind will try to trick us; our senses will lead us to the answers.

How do you get to be a proficient energy healing practitioner? Practice, practice, practice! And, never think that you know all the answers or that you know better than your client. Even the best healers I know have been mistaken at times, so it's best to be cautious. Ethics are a very important part of doing this work, so please temper the ego, practice, and trust your senses. Did I mention you should practice?

For more detailed information about the levels of the field, please refer to Barbara Brennan's book "Hands of Light."

The seven bands of the auric field can be divided between two planes: the physical and the spiritual. They are separated by the astral plane.

<u>Physical Plane</u>

Etheric Body: "I Feel Physically"

The first level of our auric field is structured. It is located between ¼ inch – one inch away from our body. This fine, blue mesh web is a blueprint of our body, including our organs. It is in constant motion as this is a state between energy and matter. The etheric structure sets up the matrix for our cells to grow. They grow along the lines of energy of the etheric matrix.

Dis-ease is expressed in tangles, breaks or disruptions in the etheric layer. This may be accompanied by a physical sensation in the area.

Personal Emotional Body: "I Feel Emotionally"

The second level is unstructured. Fluid in nature, it fluctuates between 1 – 3 inches above our body. Unlike the etheric body, the emotional body does not duplicate our physical body. Our feelings are expressed through this level.

Depending upon the emotional state, the colors can range from brilliant clear tones to dark muddy hues. Clear and energized feelings are bright and clear. Fear, grief, anger, stagnated or depleted energy may show as dark blocks of energy. Confused or muddled feelings are also dark and muddy. When we are emotionally healthy, the emotional body has all of the colors of the rainbow.

Mental Body: "I Think Clearly"

The third level of our auric field is structured. Consciousness is expressed in rational thinking and this level contains the structure of our ideas. Habitual thought patterns and attitudes get stuck here and have a profound effect on our lives.

Yellow in hue, this body is located between 3 – 8 inches above the body. It expands and becomes brighter when the person is concentrating on mental processes. Individual thoughtforms have additional colors superimposed on them, emanating from the emotional level.

Astral Body: "I Connect to Guides"

Unstructured, the fourth level is between 8 – 12 inches above the body. Relationships and emotional attachments are tethered here. The stronger the relationship, the more cords thread through this level. When relationships end, the cords are torn and need disconnection from the lower levels of the field to re-root them to the self.

People connect to each other frequently on the astral level. Compatibility often comes from connections at this level. Spiritually, our connections to angels and guides are rooted here. We receive their healing energies and this allows our soul to explore.

Spiritual Plane

Etheric Body: "Thy Will and Mine Be Done"

The fifth level of our auric field is structured. It is 1 – 2 feet above our body and supports us in manifestation by connecting our will to Spirit. It supports defining and naming things into being by connecting to Higher Will. Sound creates matter. In working with this layer, sound is most effective and may include chanting or the use of singing bowls.

This level has been described as looking like the negative of a photograph. The etheric template is the template for the etheric body, which then forms the grid structure upon which the physical body grows. Working on this level helps to support the physical template.

Expression of disease can be seen on this body as a distortion of belief and attempts to feel superior. When we are in harmony, we experience a combination of human will with a higher power.

Celestial Body: "I Love Universally"

The sixth level of our auric field is unstructured. Ranging from $2 - 2\frac{1}{2}$ feet away from the body, this level embraces a universal love for all life, not just friends and family.

This is the emotional level of the spiritual plane, where we can feel our connection to everything in the Universe, seeing light and love in all that exists. Unconditional love flows when there is a connection between our heart chakra and our celestial chakra. This body is our emotional level of the spiritual plane.

The Celestial Body been described as a beautiful iridescent ray radiating out in all directions and like the glow of a candle that warms those around us.

Ketheric Body: "I Know I Am"

This structured level is typically seen as the "beginning" or the "source" from which everything else springs. It's considered the first stage in the process of manifestation, or creation, or emanation. This is where the initial creative impulse begins.

Located 3 – 4 feet above the body, this body can expand more than 4 feet depending upon the energy of the person. It is the strongest, most resilient level of our auric field. The outer layer is like an eggshell keeping the auric field resistant to penetration and holds the entire field together.

The Ketheric Body contains a golden grid structure of all of our chakras and our physical body. It looks like thousands of golden threads intertwined around us as if we were surrounded by a golden egg-shaped mesh. It contains the life plan of this incarnation and provides our link to be one with our Creator.

Chapter Nine

Hara Line

The Hara Line is an invisible line of energy that runs from about 3 ½ feet above the head and runs through the middle of the body down through the root chakra. It resides in the auric field of our body, and exists on the level of intentionality by connecting us to our soul's purpose in this lifetime.

It is the power cord from the Universe that enlivens our physical body and, when strong, enables us to live with vitality and clarity.

Simply imagine a beam of light moving from the top of your head through your body through your root chakra and down into the ground. This is your Hara Line. When your Hara Line is in alignment, you are synchronized with the whole.

The Tan Tien is a power center in the body that gives us the impetus to move and exist. The primary center is in the second chakra and supplies the energy in our bodies to help us create the life that we wish to live. When the Tan Tien is strong and vital, we are capable of standing strong and moving forward with intention. When it is weak, we are prone to dis-ease, depression and become unmotivated.

Sometimes the Tan Tien is referred to the Golden Cauldron because it is the seat of our internal energy. It is the foundation of rooted standing, breathing, and body awareness.

Imagine a pulsing, golden light 2 ½ inches below your navel. Place your hands in the area and notice what you feel. Does it feel vibrant, powerful, strong or does it feel like it needs a boost? The Hara Line exercise in this chapter will assist in strengthening and revitalizing this area.

The Soul Seat is where our purpose in life is waiting to be unwrapped. We hold the course of our lives here and, when we open to this purpose, our lives become full, exciting and adventurous. The Hara Line runs through the Soul Seat, enlivening and waking it up.

The Soul Seat is located approximately 3 inches below the hollow of your throat. It carries the longing that leads you to accomplish your soul's purpose in this lifetime. Within it we discover everything we long to be, do, or become. Sometimes the Soul Seat is called the High Heart.

The Individuation Point is located above the head and is the spark of the beginning of this particular lifetime. It is where the physical layer of our auric field meets the God-Source, making it an important connection to fulfilling the incarnation.

This is located about 3 ½ feet above our head. Through it we have a direct connection to Spirit. It is the first point of individuation from the oneness of Spirit. The best way to describe it is that it is a small funnel that points towards the head.

<u>Hara Line Exercise</u>

I don't believe in reinventing the wheel and when I find an effective method I like to share that. This Hara Line Exercise I discovered at neozen888.wordpress.com and have found it to be the best method for aligning and strengthening the Hara Line, the Tan Tien and the Soul Seat.

Begin by standing with your feet about 3 feet apart, and bend your knees deeply until you find a comfortable stance. Let your feet turn outward to avoid twisting your knees. Take a moment to align your spine. Close your eyes if you feel comfortable doing so.

Pick up a piece of hair that is directly on top of your head. Pull it gently upwards as this will align your body on a plumb line with the earth.

Next, place the very tip of your fingers into the Tan Tien, about 2 ½ inches below your navel in the Second Chakra. Keep your fingers together, with the backs of your fingers touching. And, trust that your intention will guide you to the Tan Tien. Breathe. Hold this space for several moments.

When you are ready, move your hands into a triangle position, with your fingertips pointing down into the earth direction in front of the Tan Tien. Breathe. Focus on feeling the energies in your Tan Tien.

Bring your awareness to your upper chest area, about 3 inches below the hollow in your throat and on the midline of your body. This is your Soul Seat. Place the fingertips of both hands into this area. Again, keep your fingers together, with the backs of your fingers touching.

Imagine a sphere of diffused light that carries the longing that leads you through life to accomplish your soul's purpose. Pause for as long as you feel is needed, with slow, deep breaths.

Next, place the fingertips of your right hand into the Soul Seat and the fingertips of your left hand pointed down towards the earth, over the Tan Tien. Breathe. Feel the Hara Line running directly down from the Soul Seat through your Tan Tien, and down into the center of the earth.

After a few moments, raise the fingers of your right hand over your head. Feel the Hara Line, which extends from the Soul Seat up through your head into the Individuation Point. This is your ninth chakra. Your left hand remains at the Tan Tien for a moment.

Pause and feel the energies moving simultaneously up through your Tan Tien and down from your Individuation Point and into your Soul Seat. Breathe into this.

When you feel ready, bring your right hand to your Soul Seat with your fingers pointed up. Your left hand remains with your Tan Tien, fingers pointed down.

Feel into the Hara Line and the three points of energy. Hold your intention for the Hara Line to be straight, bright and strong. As your Hara Line aligns and strengthens, you will feel yourself aligning to your life's purpose. You may not know what it is, but you are aligned with it and your actions will automatically be synchronistic with it.

After a moment, take a deep breath and slowly release it. Bring both hands into a prayer position in front of your Soul Seat. Savor this moment and open your eyes.

<u>Healing the Hara Line Layout</u>

The purpose of this layout is to stabilize and support our center especially in times of stress and uncertainty. This technique is a synergy of what was taught at The School for Enlightenment and Healing, and Free Spirit School. I added the stone layout to assist in strengthening and revitalizing the Hara Line system.

Layout:

Ankles – Lingam – placed sideways in between

First Chakra – Black Tourmaline – placed vertically in between the legs

Torso – Large Selenite Wand – placed vertically

Fourth Chakra – Kunzite

Seventh Chakra – Selenite Wand – placed vertically above the head

Clear stones and place them on the body starting at the ankles and moving up to the crown chakra.

Before you begin, you will need to hold and stabilize your own Hara. Bend your knees a bit until they are comfortable and really feel the connection with the earth below your feet. Place your left hand at the Tan Tien with fingers facing down towards the root chakra. Place your right hand above you head with fingers pointing upwards towards the Individuation Point. Hold this pose until you feel balanced and strong. Then, slowly bring your hands together at the heart in a prayer position. Now you are ready to begin the session.

Gently pull your client's ankles to stretch legs and spine and energize the spine. You may wish to rock their legs back and forth a bit to help loosen them up. Place your thumbs on central line of client's foot just above the heal. Firmly grasp their foot with your hands.

Next, focus on your Tan Tien and Hara Line in order to create a harmonic attunement with your client's Tan Tien and Hara Line. With your intention, charge your client's Tan Tien. You are not running energy, simply working with intentionality.

Once you feel the connection, place your fingers under your client's body at the sacroiliac joint, which is where the hip bone to the sacrum, which is the triangular bone between the lumbar spine and the tailbone. Gently press and pull to the outside of the body, relaxing and expanding that joint. When you feel this area relax, repeat on the other side.

Place fingertips of both hands into the client's Tan Tien and charge until you feel a pulsing in the area. Then, point the fingers of your hand closest to the client's head towards the root and hold other hand between client's legs like you're holding a small tube until you feel a strong connection. This helps to help ground the Hara Line. Your hand should be 2 – 3 inches above the client's knees.

Next, place one hand on the Tan Tien and one on the Soul Seat. This is located in the breastbone, a long flat bone in the central part of the chest. Run energy for a few moments until you feel the client is ready for the next step.

Move your hand closest to the client's feet to the Soul Seat with fingers pointing into the breastbone. Hold your other hand about a half-inch above the client's head like you're holding a tube at Individuation Point until you feel a strong energetic connection. Concentrate on your own Individuation Point and Hara Line at the same time.

Next, place both hands to the client's Soul Seat. Expand your client's entire essence by imagining you and your client moving into the fourth level of their auric field for a few minutes. Hold this feeling until you feel this expansion complete.

To end the session, remove the stones starting at the crown and moving down to the ankles. Take a moment to clear the stones.

Then, gently rake the body beginning at the shoulders and arms and moving down the torso and the legs. Hold the client's ankles and once again pull the legs. You may also want to gently shake or rock the client's legs.

After this, have your client sit up. Rub their arms, back and legs until they are fully aware and back in their body.

Chapter Ten

DaEL Walker's Crystal Healing Technique

In the first crystal class I took in 1991, we studied the techniques in DaEl Walker's Crystal Healing Book. DaEl Walker was the Founder of the Crystal Awareness Institute, an incredible teacher and lecturer, and Crystalotherapy Master Healer. For over 25 years, he focused his research on subtle energy, crystals, healing, and sensitivity training, and was one of the world's leading authorities on crystal skulls.

I met DaEl in 2011 when he came to Free Spirit Crystals to conduct workshops and healing sessions. His depth of knowledge of crystals and heart-felt teaching style touched everyone who attended his classes each time that he came to Milwaukee. DaEl and I established a lovely rapport and, when I told him I wanted to include the crystal wand healing technique in my book, he graciously agreed. He and I have the same philosophy that this work should be shared to everyone for the good of all.

DaEl's crystal wand healing technique is the most effective crystal procedure that I have learned. I love it for its simplicity and for its many uses. This approach can be used for aches, pains, strains, bruises, sprains, burns, headaches, broken bones, balancing systems of the body, centering and meditation. It uses the principle that crystals have the closest vibration to that of the human body and, when you place the crystals on the body, it allows the body to heal itself naturally.

All you need for this technique are two polished clear quartz crystal wands. The wands should have a rounded base at the bottom and a termination on the top. It is important that you use polished crystals as you will be placing them directly on the skin. Unpolished crystals have very sharp edges that can cause cuts.

I use DaEl's balancing technique before every session I conduct. It not only balances the nervous system, circulatory system and brain but it also allows the client to become calm and relaxed. When the body is in a state of relaxation, it allows the energy to move through with ease giving the body more access for healing. I consider it to be the most useful technique that I have ever learned, and strongly urge everyone who uses crystals to learn it as well.

<u>Balancing Technique</u>

This approach covers three areas of the body – the nervous system, the circulatory system, and the brain. It's best if you have a massage table for your client to lie on for both you and your client's comfort. If your client cannot lie on a table, this technique can be done sitting in a chair.

When DaEl devised this healing technique, he understood that the crystals needed to be cleared before using them. He tested out several invocations until he came up with the following saying and found that this was the most effective: *I invoke the Light of the Christ within. I am a clear and perfect channel. Light is my guide.*

This invocation is repeated three times, either silently in your mind or out loud. Say this before you begin the healing to clear the crystals, when you place the crystals on the body to activate a five-minute cycle and when you are finished.

The invocation not only clears the crystals but it amplifies the energy to make them more powerful for the balancing and healing. DaEl discovered that the greatest flow of energy lasted five minutes after saying the Light Invocation. Thus, with this technique, the crystals are held at each area for five minutes. If you feel the need to keep the crystals in one place for longer than five minutes, simply repeat the Light Invocation again three times.

I have replaced the word 'Christ' with 'Universal Energy.' Some practitioners say the Light of God, others use Buddha, Quan Yin, or any other enlightened Master Teacher. The effect is the same.

This balancing technique begins by having your client lie on the table. Stand at the foot of the table with a polished quartz healing wand in each hand. The crystal in your left hand will have the termination facing the wrist. The crystal in your right hand will have the termination facing the fingertips. This is because the energy of the body moves from left to right. The blood flows into the heart from the left and leaves from the right. It is the natural flow of the body.

Center and ground yourself so that you are fully present for your client. Say the Light Invocation three times to clear the crystals. Next, place the left-hand crystal flush on the bottom of your client's left foot and the right-hand crystal flush on the bottom of their right foot. This is the nervous system balancing.

Next, say the Light Invocation to activate a five-minute cycle and hold the crystals steady for the duration of the balancing. After five minutes, remove the crystals from the bottoms of the feet and go to the hip area. Find the indented area right below the hip bone on each side of the hips, and place one crystal point facing in on one hip, and one crystal point facing out at the other. Both terminations should be going in the same direction. This is the circulatory balancing.

Repeat the Light Invocation three times to activate the five-minute cycle. After five minutes, slowly remove the crystals from the hips.

Next move to the top of the client's head. Place the left-handed point facing the wrist and the right-handed crystal facing the fingertips. Gently place the crystals on either side of the head near the temples so as not to cause discomfort. This is the brain balancing.

Repeat the Light Invocation three times to activate the five-minute cycle. When you are finished, slowly remove the crystals from the sides of the head and clear them by saying the Light Invocation three times.

This can be the completion of your session, or you can go on to do other healing modalities after this such as Reiki, Healing Touch, a crystal layout or any other of the techniques in this book.

Note: You do not have to clear the crystals each time you move from place to place as you are working on the same client. Clear them before and after the session.

There are seven steps to each five-minute cycle:

- Calm

- Tingling

- Uneven Pulsing

- Heat

- Cool

- Heat

- Even Pulse/Calm

You may not sense these, or they may manifest unevenly as the energy moves from the crystals and into your client. It doesn't matter if you feel the stages or not because they are working regardless. It takes some people a bit of practice to feel this while others sense it immediately. Your client may also feel the different stages or you may feel them together. Practice, practice, practice!!

You can also do this balancing on yourself. Many people do it daily to energize their systems.

Chapter Eleven

Crystal Wand Healing Techniques

If you have a situation where you simply want to use the crystals to help heal a part of the body, it is not mandatory to begin by doing the fifteen-minute balancing. I take my stones with me wherever I go just in case I have crystal emergency!

Here is a very simple exercise that I show my students so that they can work on themselves and others, if needed.

Begin by asking the person where they would like you to place the crystals. This consent is very important. Most people will intuitively know where they need help.

Place the left-hand crystal with the point facing the wrist and the right-hand crystal with the point facing the fingertips.

Next, clear your crystals by repeating the Light Invocation three times: *I invoke the light of Universal Energy within. I am a clear and perfect channel. Light is my guide.*

Place the crystals on opposite sides of the pain. For example, if the person has a headache, the crystals will be place on both sides of the head. If the person had a sore foot, place one crystal on the top and one crystal on the bottom of the foot. If the person has a sore back, place one crystal on the front of the body and the other crystal on the back, and so forth. This allows a cycle of energy to rotate around the area in order to align, balance and bring the body back to its natural vibration.

Hold the crystals on the area for five minutes. If you feel the need to hold them there longer, you can say the Light Invocation every five minutes to reset the cycle. Stay on an area as long as you'd like as long as you say the invocation every five minutes for optimal effect.

When you are finished, slowly remove the crystals and say the Light Invocation to clear them. The reason you need to remove the crystals slowly is because you are working in an electromagnetic field. If you snap the crystals away, it interferes with the flow of the field.

For chronic problems, you can repeat this several times per day until the person finds relief. Know that the crystals are not only working on the physical body, but the etheric, mental and emotional bodies as well. This helps to promote healing the whole system, not just a symptom.

Again, you can do this technique on yourself and repeat it as often as you'd like. I have used it on my sprained ankle, fractured wrist, body aches, sore knees and cuts.

<u>Laser Wands</u>

Laser wands are rather rugged looking crystals that are tapered and come to a very distinct, sharp termination. They are reminiscent of Lemurian crystals with hieroglyphics on the sides, containing knowledge of ancient healing techniques. Laser crystals also have the following aspects:

Direct, well focused energy

Open chakras

Helps clear negativity from rooms

Promote a spirit of oneness and love

Create protective barriers

Perform psychic surgery

Direct connection to the soul; access information concerning the soul's journey

Level of the Field Healing with a Laser Wand and Stones

This healing assists with breaking up blockages in the seven levels of the auric field before they can filter down into the physical body. These blockages can be emotional, environmental toxins, or negative outside influences. By using a laser wand, you can detect these influences and block them, slow their progress or eliminate them altogether. Use the laser wand to draw out blockages, remove impediments, do 'etheric surgery,' cleanse the area, and patch holes in the field.

It is important that, before doing work with laser wands, you become very familiar with working in the levels of the field. This includes practicing feeling the etheric energy of many people before including a laser wand in your healing work. You are looking for differences in the auric field's temperature, a mushy feeling, a snag, a tear, interference in the energy flow, bumpiness – anything that does not feel like a smooth flow of energy.

The purposes of using stones when doing a level of the field healing include:

- Strengthen and protect each level

- Break up blocks in the physical body and the etheric layers

- Expedite the search for snarls, breaks and interference in the field

<u>Healing Session</u>

Begin the session by holding the client's ankles until you feel like you are connected to their energy. You will feel a sort of oneness with your client and a bond from your heart to theirs.

Once you feel that bond, begin to feel into the levels of the field using the laser wand sideways as a guide. This is simply an exploration to help you assess what is happening in the field. After assessing the client's field, choose from the suggested list of stones for your layout:

First Chakra
Black Tourmaline, Elestial, Lingams

Second Chakra
Bronzite, Labradorite, Tiger eye

Third Chakra
Citrine, Malachite, Amber

Fourth Chakra
Kunzite, Morganite, Hiddenite

Fifth Chakra
Chrysocolla, Aquamarine, Dumortierite

Sixth Chakra
Azurite, Herkimer Diamond, Apophyllite Pyramid

Seventh Chakra
Quartz Cluster, Rutilated Quartz, Selenite

Anywhere
Nuummite, Shungite, Galena

Tools for Healing

Laser Wand, Selenite Wand

Begin by clearing the stones, then place them on your client's body beginning at their root chakra and moving up to the crown. Next, go back into the levels of the field and search for whatever imbalances might be there. It takes as long as it takes, so do not rush the process. Remember that you are responsible for the person on the table, and do not want to do anything sudden or rash. This is their energy field that you are in, so please take that responsibility seriously.

When you find a snag or interference, gently use the Laser Wand to cut through it as if you are doing surgery. Feel into the suture and 'look' for anything that you feel needs to be removed, such as a sliminess, something that feels hard, a feeling of cracked glass. There are many ways to feel things and that is why you must practice working with as many people's fields as possible before you do this work. I can't emphasize enough the need to practice this technique before using laser wands.

When you feel like you have removed the interference, you will use the laser wand to suture the incision just as a surgeon would. Imagine you have a thread on the tip of the wand and sew up the slit you have created. Then, place the laser wand on top of the area to run light into it so as to 'heal' the incision. Repeat this throughout all seven levels until you feel that the energy is light and flowing.

If you do not sense anything at all, there is no need to do any auric fieldwork. Simply do energy work on the physical body. Or, you can do energy work on the client after you have completed your exploration and work in the levels of the field.

When you have completed the work in the levels of the field, remove and clear the stones beginning at the crown chakra. Then, use a Selenite Wand to clear and fluff each layer of the auric field starting at the 7th level and working down to the first level. Selenite has a very fast and light energy that helps to restore resilience in the aura.

To end the session, hold the ankles and bring your client's energy into your hands in order to ensure that they are awake and aware. When they slowly sit up, rub their arms, legs and back to help them feel their body and become grounded.. Look into their eyes – if they have a faraway look, continue to gently rub them until they are clear and bright. You can have them hold a sizeable piece of hematite or black tourmaline to help them with the grounding process. Often I will offer them a glass of water, a cracker or a cookie to make sure they are fully functioning before they leave.

<u>Vogel and 12-Sided Crystals</u>

Vogel crystals were created by Marcel Vogel. Vogel was a scientist who worked for IBM for 27 years and is responsible for over one hundred scientific patents. In order to measure the energy that a crystal was putting out, Vogel developed a radionic device known as the Omega 5. This instrument measured energies beyond what was currently capable with standardized scientific equipment.

After retirement from IBM in 1984, Vogel started Psychic Research Inc. where he conducted original research into advanced crystal technologies and created the 12-sided Vogel crystal cut. It is based on the pattern of the "Tree of Life" and is more energetic and focused often being compared to a laser beam.

The larger tip of the crystal is called the male side or the firing tip and the tapered end is known as the female side or the receptor. These crystals have very focused, direct energy and they work to restructure the body.

The Vogel crystal is a very specific cut and quite expensive. There are only a few people in the world who cut authentic Vogel crystals – the rest are manufactured mostly in Brazil. However, I have had great success using plain 12-sided crystals (which are not considered to be Vogel) as they have a very direct focus and are wonderful for opening up lines of light in the body and balancing the spine.

Besides the three techniques listed below, you can also use them in psychic surgery on the levels of the field.

According to Marcel:

The crystal is a quantum converter that is able to transmit energy in a form that has discreet biological effects. This is most likely a resonant effect. The human body, on an energetic level, is an array of oscillating points that are layered and have a definite symmetry and structure. This crystallinity is apparent on both a subtle energetic or quantum level as well as the macro level. The bones, tissues, cells, and fluids of the body have a definite crystallinity about them. The structure of the fluids, cells, and tissues of the body tends to become unstructured or incoherent when dis-ease or distress is present. The physical body is comprised of liquid crystal systems in the cell membranes, intercellular fluids, as well as larger structures such as the fatty tissues, muscular and nervous systems, lymph, blood, and so on.[2]

---

[2] http://wwwmarcelvogel.org/

<u>Joint Energy Healing</u>

This technique opens up lines of light between joints in order to relax and rejuvenate the joints. You will need two 12-sided clear quartz crystals.

Begin by clearing the crystals by saying the Light Invocation three times. Beginning at the left shoulder, draw a counterclockwise circle around the shoulder joint to open the energy flow and then place the male side of the crystal directly on the joint.

With the second crystal, draw a counterclockwise circle around the elbow joint to open the energy flow. Place the male side of the second crystal on the elbow joint facing down towards the wrist to allow the energy to flow through the female tip. Hold the crystals here until you feel a free and easy flow of energy between the joints.

Run energy from the top crystal to the bottom crystal. Occasionally take the bottom crystal and run a line of energy from the shoulder to the elbow. This also helps to open and clear the area.

Next, remove the crystals and draw a clockwise circle around the shoulder and elbow joints to close the areas.

Draw a counterclockwise circle around the elbow and place the male side of the crystal on the elbow joint. Draw a counterclockwise circle around the wrist and place the male side of the second crystal on the wrist facing down towards the fingertips to allow the energy to flow through the female tip. Again, hold the crystals here until you feel a free and easy flow between the joints. Occasionally take the bottom crystal and run a line of energy from the elbow to the wrist..

Remove the crystals and draw a clockwise circle around the elbow and wrist joints. Open the wrist joint by drawing counterclockwise over it. Place the male side on the wrist pointing towards the fingers. Using the second crystal, draw lines of light three times from the wrist down each corresponding fingertip until you've done the entire hand. Draw clockwise around the wrist to close it.

Now go to the hip and draw counterclockwise in this area. Place the male side of the crystal on the hip and repeat the process as before this time opening the area at the bottom of the knee and placing the male side of the second crystal here pointing down towards the ankle. You may take the bottom crystal and run a line of light from the hip to the knee to expedite the energy flow. Again, hold them in this position until you feel a free and easy flow of energy. Remove the crystals and draw counterclockwise circles around each joint.

Place the male side of the top crystal below the knee joint and repeat the process, placing the male side of the second crystal on the bottom of the ankle joint with the female side facing down to allow for the release of energy. Again, hold them in this position until you feel a free and easy flow of energy. Occasionally take the bottom crystal and run a line of energy from the knee to the ankle.

Remove the crystals and draw a clockwise circle around the knee and ankle.

Open the ankle joint by drawing counterclockwise and then place the male side on the lower part of the ankle with the other point facing the feet. Using the second crystals, draw lines of light from the ankle out to the end of each toe. Do this three times per toe. Draw clockwise over the ankle to close it.

Repeat this process on the other side.

After completion of the entire procedure, place your hands on each joint starting at the shoulders holding them there for a minute or two. Continue this process until you have held each joint. Finish by holding the ankles helping to ground your client.

<u>Vertebral Healing with 12-Sided Quartz</u>

This technique is wonderful for arthritis, lower back pain, and stiffness in the back and neck as well as providing a relaxing experience. It balances the spine and opens up energy blocks in the vertebrae. You will need two 12-sided quartz crystals for this healing.

Begin by having your client lie face down on the table preferably with a face cradle to make the neck more comfortable. Place your hands on the upper back and run energy into the back. Gently push your hands back and forth to massage, relax, open and soften the area. Continue the procedure down the entire back until you feel it is ready to receive the crystal energy.

Using the male end of the 12 sided quartz, begin at the first vertebrae at the top of the client's spine and place the tips of the crystals on each side of the vertebrae. Hold it there until you feel area has taken in all the energy it can. Continue working down each vertebra in the same manner. Do not use a lot of pressure when pointing the crystals into the skin; gently place them there as these crystals can feel like needles!

When you have completed the crystal restoration, use your fingertips to massage the sides of each vertebrae individually until you have completed all of them. When you are done, place your hands on the upper back and working down running energy and massaging each area.

Lightly rake the back and the legs completing the session by holding the bottoms of the feet until your client feels ready to get up.

Chapter Twelve

Crystal Healing for Crystal Practitioners

Placing stones on and around our bodies invites their vibrational energy to permeate down into our physical being. The energy of the stones sifts down into our organs, bones, tissues, blood stream and structures of our bodies in order to help align it to a more perfect union.

Layouts aid in relaxation, mindfulness, awareness and release. I encourage people to journal their experiences after each layout and keep a log of their progress. Remember, all healing is not physical. Sometimes the most important healing occurs on an awareness level so that we may release what no longer serves us and move into a life free of emotional bondage.

I composed my first layout, Initiation Layout, in 1994, after meditating with crystals. I was told that this would be the first of a trio of layouts to be used in succession. After the Initiation Layout, came the Release Layout, and finally the Integration Layout, all of which are used in our classes. Little was I to know that almost two hundred layouts would follow, each dealing with a specific situation.

Just a reminder: always start laying stones at the feet and work your way up. The last step is to add stones to your hands, if included in the layout. Either listen to a guided meditation or lay silently for about 20 minutes. At the end, remove the stones from your head first and down to the bottoms of your feet. Remove stones in your hands last. And, if possible, journal about what you experienced.

I am going to include the three layouts that I just mentioned as they are wonderful for starting you on a path to inner healing. I have found that using them in succession is very helpful in opening your body, mind and spirit to begin a renewed way of living. I suggest that you use each one several times a week for one week and then go to the next. Please keep a journal of what you experience as this will be a helpful reference for you as you continue your journey.

If you are interested in more of my layouts, please refer to The KISS Guide to Stone Layouts and The KISS Guide to More Stone Layouts.

<u>Initiation Layout</u>

The purpose of the Initiation Layout is to bring each person's spirit back to it's beginning, to start over on its way to finding itself. It is designed to awaken each center to its own power unaffected by outside conditioning and beliefs therefore allowing for the opening of living with all possibilities. It is to empty out the old way of living while making the transition to knowing one's pure essence.

Layout:

Below Feet - Laser Wand and Selenite wand (points toward the feet)

First Chakra - Terminated Black Tourmaline (with termination towards root chakra)

Second Chakra - Labradorite

Third Chakra - Citrine Point or Golden or White Calcite Rhomboid
(angled with points toward heart and sacral chakra)

Fourth Chakra - Morganite

Fifth Chakra -Aquamarine

Sixth Chakra - Pietersite

Seventh Chakra –Laser Wand and Selenite wand
(points toward the head)

Hands - Labradorite

Start doing some deep breathing, lay with your eyes closed and relax for 20 minutes. If possible, write down impressions of your session after it's over.

<u>Release Layout</u>

The release layout is designed to help you let go of unwanted negative energy, old belief systems and confusion. It will assist in clearing out the energy structure of the body in order to allow new and clear thoughts, feelings and beliefs to enter.

Layout:

Below Feet – Obsidian Sphere

Feet – Selenite

First Chakra – Black Tourmaline

Second Chakra– Ruby

Third Chakra – Kunzite

Fourth Chakra– Malachite

Fifth Chakra – Azurite

Sixth Chakra – Selenite

Seventh Chakra – Selenite

Hands – Selenite

Lay with the layout for a minimum of twenty minutes and then journal what you experienced.

<u>Integration Layout</u>

The integration layout is designed to assist in integrating the conflicting feelings, which reside inside of each of us. It helps to connect each area of the body to body, mind and spirit in order to have a feeling of wholeness and well-being. It is used to aid in clarification of confusing thought patterns and inner turmoil.

Layout:

At the feet – Two Smoky Quartz points, one at each foot, pointing toward the foot

First Chakra – Black Tourmaline

Second chakra – Carnelian

Third Chakra – Amber

Fourth Chakra – Rhodochrosite, Kunzite, Rhodonite

Fifth Chakra – Turquoise

Sixth Chakra – Sugilite

Above Head - Quartz crystal pointing toward crown

Hands – Mochi Marbles

Lay for 20 minutes once a day for as long as necessary. If possible, do a guided visualization in your body about integrating the various parts of you, which seem to be in dispute.

<u>Balancing Organs of the Second and Third Chakras</u>

Our organs have a substantial responsibility to maintain the functionality of the body. Each of them has their own, unique system that works in unity with the others. When one is not operating at its full capacity, it affects the flow and workings of all the other systems of the body.

This technique assists the organs of the Second and Third Chakras to function in the most energetic way that they can while bringing balance and flow to the entire body. You will need two quartz healing wands for the layout for this technique. Each of the stones in the layout is specific for the organ upon which it is placed.

Layout:

Bottoms of feet – small Laser Wands pointing downwards

Middle of legs – Black Tourmaline with striations parallel to the legs

Second Chakra – Moonstone (One large or several small)

Gall Bladder – Malachite

Bladder, Stomach, Liver, Spleen – Bloodstones

Kidneys – Seraphinite

Pancreas – Rose Quartz

Fourth Chakra – Chrysoprase

Fifth Chakra – Chrysocolla

Sixth Chakra – Amethyst

Seventh Chakra – Fluorite

Hands – Red Jasper

Before you begin, palpate the feet, legs, hips, and the second and third chakras to introduce a calmness and sense of security to the body.

Move to the client's spleen, hold a quartz healing wand directly on the area with the point facing downward towards the second chakra. Hold the quartz until you feel a flow of energy pulsating in your hand.

Next, point the quartz down towards the spleen, draw a counter-clockwise circle around the organ, draw the energy up and flick it either towards the sky or down into the ground. Repeat this three times and then draw clock-wise around the area and once again place the crystal directly on the organ with the point facing the second chakra for about a half minute. Repeat this on the stomach, pancreas, liver, gallbladder, intestines and bladder.

Next, place your hand with the crystal flush underneath the left kidney area with the crystal point facing towards the second chakra. Place your other hand on the top of the body and hold this position for at least two minutes. Repeat on the right kidney. Using a quartz healing wand in each hand, place one crystal close to the groin area on each leg (make sure you are not touching any private areas) with the points facing down towards the feet. This allows the energy of the entire healing to radiate downward and solidify it. Hold the crystals here for a minimum of two minutes. Grounding is a very important step at the end of this healing as it helps to maintain balance in the entire system.

Remove the stones beginning at the head and going down to the feet. To end the session, repeat the palpations and then gently rake the energy field including the body.

<u>Brain Healing Method</u>

This brain healing incorporates the hand positions that I have experimented with over the past 20 years and I have found to be very effective when working on the head.

Here is a basic, calming chakra layout that is balancing for the entire body as well as the brain. In addition to the stones, two crystal healing wands are required.

No stones are needed on the sixth or seventh chakras as you will be working in this area. Let's cover all the bases!

Layout:

Between ankles – Lingam

Between knees – Black Tourmaline

Second Chakra – Moonstone

Third Chakra – Mica Lepidolite

Fourth Chakra – Rose Quartz

Fifth Chakra – Sodalite

Begin by doing a 15-minute crystal balancing on the feet, hips and heads. When you have finished the balancing put the crystals away and go to the top of the head.

Place both hands under the neck, also known as the Mouth of God, and very gently begin to massage the neck. This allows your client to relax and let go.

Using your subtle sense perception, pinpoint places in the head area which seem hard, stiff or rigid and, using your fingertips, send lines of light into those areas. Gently place your fingertips on the occipital ridge and run energy. I usually keep my fingers here for a few minutes as it is very comforting and helps to open up the spinal cord.

Begin to move your fingers up from the occipital ridge to behind the ears, massaging the backs of the ears. Do this several times. Lightly massage the ears themselves, and then move on to the cheeks and jaw in a roundabout motion for a minute or two.

Place your fingertips right below the cheekbones and place your thumbs below the jaw. Run energy through your hands into the area for a couple of minutes. Then, gently massage the temples for a few minutes.

Gently place your fingertips on the bones directly below the eyes. Place your thumbs on the hairline. Run energy for a couple of minutes, then gently massage the forehead.

Place your fingertips directly above the eyebrows and your thumbs on the crown for a couple of minutes. Next, gently massage the crown and the back of the head for a minute or two.

Place your fingertips on the hairline and your thumbs on the crown for a couple of minutes. Next, place your fingertips on the temples and your thumbs on the back the head running energy back and forth between the temples. Notice if there is a clear path between the two or if it feels like there is a block. Continue to do this until if feels clear.

Next, move your hands to the sides of the head for a few minutes. Then, place one hand under the neck and the other on the heart. Hold this for a couple of minutes.

When you feel that the client is ready, gently remove the stones from the body beginning at the throat chakra. Remove the grounding stones last. Clear the stones.

From here, you will gently rake the body with your fingertips beginning at the shoulders and working your way down the body. Then, move to the client's feet and hold the bottoms of the feet until your client begins to wake up.

Have your client sit up and then rub their arms, legs, back and shoulders to get them back into their body.

Lymph System Drainage

According to Livescience.com, the lymphatic system is "a network of tissues and organs that help rid the body of toxins, waste and other unwanted materials. The primary function of the lymphatic system is to transport lymph, a fluid containing infection-fighting white blood cells, throughout the body."[3]

There are hundreds of lymph nodes throughout the body which need to stay clear and healthy in order for our bodies to maintain optimum health. Our tonsils, adenoids, spleen, and thymus are all a part of the lymphatic system.

This procedure will assist the flow of lymph throughout the body in order to eliminate toxins. Please be sure to drink sufficient amounts of water after having this technique done on you. In addition to the layout stones, you will need two quartz healing wands.

---

[3] Zimmermann, K. A. (2018, February 21). Lymphatic System: Facts, Functions & Diseases. Retrieved from https://www.livescience.com/26983-lymphatic-system.html

Layout:

Bottoms of Feet – Selenite Wands

Inside and Outside of the Legs – Selenite Wands

Pelvic Area – Chlorite Crystals or Tumbled Seraphinite

Spleen – Red Jasper

Thymus Gland – Lapis Lazuli

Fifth Chakra – Turquoise

Along Side Body – Selenite Wands

Hands – Seraphinite

Begin by doing the 15 minute crystal wand balancing found in chapter 10. Using a quartz healing wand, begin at one side of the throat by drawing counter-clockwise circles around the cervical lymph nodes on the side of the client's neck. Pull the crystal away from the body and release it to the ground with a flick of your wrist. Repeat this six times and then draw a clockwise circle around the area to close it. Repeat on the other side of the client's neck.

Move the quartz healing wand to the upper part of the client's chest. This is where the thoracic duct and thymus gland are located. Draw counter-clockwise around the area, pull the crystal away from the body and release the negative energies into the ground. Repeat six times. When complete, draw a clockwise circle around the area.

Continue to the client's upper arms. Draw counter-clockwise circles under the armpit and then move the crystal down the arm to release the energy out of the fingertips to assist the flow of the axillary lymph nodes. Do this five times(one time for each finger) on each side, drawing a clockwise circle around the armpits to close the area.

Next, place the crystal directly on the client's spleen. This is located under the rib cage next to the stomach on the left side of the client's abdomen. Hold it there for a minute or two to help strengthen the energy of the spleen. Then, again draw counter-clockwise six times at the spleen and flick the crystal towards the earth. Draw a clockwise circle around the area to close it.

At the pelvic area, draw a counterclockwise circle around the area and then direct the crystal point down the leg to the knee and flick the crystal down towards the earth. Remember to do this six times, close the area with a clockwise motion and then repeat on the other side.

At the knee, direct the crystal point down the leg to the toes, and direct the energy out, one toe at a time. Do this five times, one for each toe, then repeat on the other side.

Remove the stones starting at the upper body and clear them. To end the session, take your fingertips and gently rake the entire lymph system until you sense an even flow. Then place your hands underneath the ankles and very gently shake the legs back and forth to assist in circulating the lymph.

Emotional Awareness Technique

The purpose of this technique is to gently draw out suppressed feelings which have been compacted over years of silence and compliance. This healing is designed to unlock the feeling and allow a recognition and ultimate release of their emotions.

In addition to the layout stones, you will need a Rose Quartz Point and Selenite wand. Have a notebook and pen handy to transcribe any thoughts and feelings your client wishes to express during the session so that they can use it as a reference when they leave.

Reminder: this is not a counseling session. The information is solely for your client's benefit to assist them in understanding the feelings that they have been suppressing. Your job is to provide a safe haven for them to feel and express themselves. You may suggest that your client visit a licensed therapist to assist them in moving through their feelings.

Layout:

Between ankles – Lingam laying sideways

Between legs – Smoky Elestial

Thighs – Petrified Wood

Second Chakra – Orange Calcite

Third Chakra – Honey Calcite

Fourth Chakra – Rose Quartz

Fifth Chakra – Chrysocolla

Sixth Chakra – Ametrine

Seventh Chakra – Golden Calcite Rhomboid

Hands - Azurite

To begin, clear stones and place them on the client beginning at the ankles and moving upward. Then, hold the bottoms of the feet and invite your client to bring their energy to your hands. When you feel that they have met you there, begin a brief chelation or palpation beginning at the feet and moving upwards towards the head. This should take no longer than ten minutes. It allows your client to relax and the energy in the body to connect.

After this, hold the rose quartz on or above your client's heart chakra and allow that energy to gradually sink down into the area. The crystal should be pointing towards the chin to allow a flow of communication from their heart to their throat. After a few minutes, ask your client what they are feeling and where they are feeling it in their body.

Give them time to respond as sometimes it takes a bit for some people to access their feelings.

When your client has responded, ask them to check inside their heart for any information about the feelings, i.e. – where is it coming from, is there a situation that corresponds with this feeling, what are they learning from this feeling or situation. Take a moment to write down the information that is forth coming from your client so that they can use it later as a reference for personal growth and understanding.

Do NOT react or respond to what your client is relaying. You are just holding a safe space for them to feel. It is not your job to be the therapist. Write down what they are saying so that they can refer to it later with a therapist.

When your client feels like they have a clear picture of the meaning of this feeling, lay your hand on the heart chakra to fill it with light.

Repeat this with the third and then the second chakras by holding the rose quartz on or above your client's chakra and allow that energy to gradually sink down into the area. Remember, the crystal should be pointing towards the chin to allow a flow of communication from the chakra to the throat. Allow your client ample time to describe what they are feeling in their body and take some time to write this down for your client.

When your client is comfortable ending the session, remove the stones beginning with the crown chakra and clear them. Then, gently stroke the client's arms, hands, legs and feet.

Finally, sweep the levels of the auric field with the Selenite wand beginning at the first level and ending at the seventh to provide a safe boundary for them to come back into the space. After the client sits up, rub their back, arms and legs to bring them back and ground them.

<u>Heart Healing with Stones</u>

This healing is designed to assist in finding the place inside of ourselves which can sustain our own self love and compassion. It is to aid in the discovery of the child within who needs care, attention and soothing. This layout and healing will help in bringing up feelings which have been buried since early childhood so that they can be released thus allowing for a more sustained feeling of inner joy.

Layout:

Feet – Rose Quartz

First Chakra – Emerald

Second Chakra – Rhodonite

Third Chakra – Aventurine

Fourth Chakra – Kunzite

Fifth Chakra – Chrysoprase

Sixth Chakra – Rhodochrosite

Seventh Chakra – Rose Quartz Point Facing Down

Hands – Rose Quartz

Begin by clearing the stones and then placing them on the client, starting at the feet and moving up to the crown chakra.

Hold the rose quartz which are at the feet directly on the feet and allow that energy to rise up into the legs. When you feel that the energy has reached the second chakra, place the stones back to the bottoms of the feet.

Next, move to the second chakra and place one hand on top and one hand underneath the body as to embrace the client. Hold this position until it feels right to move, then do the same on the third and fourth chakras.

Move to the client's shoulder and cradle first one arm, and then move to the other side and cradle the other. Then, place your hands on the shoulders and hold this for a moment. When you are ready, place one hand underneath the neck and the other on the heart. Pause as long as you feel is right.

Gently move your hands so that your fingertips are under the occipital ridge and cradle the head. Hold this position for as long as you feel is right.

Then, remove the stones starting at the crown chakra and moving down. Clear the stones. Finish the healing by lightly stroking the client beginning at the shoulders and working your way to the feet. When the sit up, rub their arms, back and legs until they are fully awake.

<u>Inflammation Reduction Healing Technique</u>

The basis of this technique is to use a variety of stones in order to pinpoint and allow for the body to release inflammation. While much inflammation is located in the joints, this procedure also assists with swelling in the organs to help regulate and assimilate the body's entire functioning systems. When inflammation is under control, the capacity of the body to maintain health is increased.

You will need two additional pieces of Malachite and two quartz crystal healing wands for this session.

Layout:

Bottoms of Feet – Crystal Points, points facing downward

Between Legs – Two Smoky Quartz Points, points facing downward

First Chakra – Green Calcite

Second Chakra – Orange Calcite

Third Chakra, Liver and Spleen – Malachite

Fourth Chakra – Green Calcite

Fifth Chakra – Turquoise

Sixth Chakra – Azurite

Hands – Malachite

Begin by holding Malachite on the feet for approximately five minutes until you feel a draw of energy coming down into the soles of the feet. Then, move to the client's shoulders and place a piece of malachite on each shoulder. Hold two quartz healing wands on the upper arm sandwiching the arm with the crystals with the points facing the elbow. Hold this until you feel a release in the shoulder and energy moving down the arm.

Next, place the Malachite in the elbow area and place the healing wands below the elbow, sandwiching the arm between the stones. Again, wait for a release in the elbow and a flow of energy going towards the hand.

Move to the client's wrist and place the malachite on the wrist, sandwich the crystals on the top and inner hand. Wait for the release and flow of energy. Repeat this on the other side for the shoulder, elbow and wrist.

Place one crystal on the right side of the rib cage and the other on the left side of the rib cage with the points facing downwards. Hold until for a few minutes or until you feel an even flow of energy going down the body. Repeat this on the sides of the second chakra and at the hips.

Next, place a Malachite on the right knee. Sandwich the crystals on the legs directly below the knee. Once again, feel for a release in the knee and a flow of energy moving down the leg.

Move the Malachite under the Achilles heel and hold the crystals on either side of the ankles with the points facing downward. Wait for the release and flow of energy.

Hold the malachite on the top of the foot and a healing crystal on the bottom of the foot until you feel a release and flow of energy.

Move to the other side of the client's body. Place the Malachite on the left knee. Sandwich the crystals on the legs directly below the knee. Once again, feel for a release in the knee and a flow of energy moving down the leg.

Move the Malachite under the Achilles heel and the crystals on either side of the ankles. Wait for the release and flow of energy.

Hold the Malachite on the top of the foot and a healing crystal on the bottom of the foot until you feel a release and flow of energy.

To end the session, remove the stones starting at the sixth chakra and moving down the body to remove the Smoky Quartz last. Briefly place your hands on each joint that you worked on and gently massage the arms, torso, legs and feet. Give your client a glass of water, and have them hold Hematite to get them become grounded when the session is over.

<u>Mind Calming with Stones</u>

With this particular practice, we will use stones over the entire body as our mind is not just in our head, but in every nerve and every cell. When we are able to calm the nervous system and the cellular body, the brain calming will be even more effective.

Because so many of us are conditioned to think more than feel, we will use several grounding stones to assist the client in shifting the focus of energy from the head to the root chakra. Staying grounded and centered gives the brain permission to slow down the thoughts and become more serene.

The rest of the chakra stones will assist in calming and creating a more even flow of energy throughout the body. In addition to the stones, you will need a Selenite wand.

Layout:

In Between Ankles – Lingam placed sideways

In Between Legs at the Knee – Black Tourmaline

Thighs – Black Kyanite

Second Chakra – Moonstone

Under the Adrenal Glands – Mica Lepidolite

Third Chakra – Large Mica Lepidolite

Fourth Chakra – Kunzite

Fifth Chakra – Lapis Lazuli

Sixth Chakra – Fluorite

Hands – Mochi Marbles

Clear the stones and place the stones on the body beginning at the feet and root first in order to maintain as much grounding as possible throughout the session.

Begin by placing your hands under the neck and allow your client to relax into them. Then, place your fingertips gently on the occipital ridge and lightly massage the area. Continue until you feel time to move to the next step.

When you are ready, place one hand on the back of the neck, and the other on the heart. Stay here for a few minutes, then place your hands on the client's shoulders. Hold this position for a couple of minutes.

Move one hand on the top of the stomach and the other hand underneath the stomach, again holding this until it feels right to move on. Place one hand on top of the second chakra and the other underneath. Pause, then move to the client's hips and place one hand on each.

Move one hand on the top of the left thigh and the other underneath. Hold this position until it feels right, then move one hand on top of the knee and the other underneath. After a moment, place one hand on top of the lower leg and the other underneath.

Move to the client's other side and repeat the process by placing one hand on the top of the right thigh and one underneath. Pause, and then continue to the knee and lower leg. Pause to hold the client's ankles for a moment, then place your hands on the bottoms of the feet. Hold your hands in place until it feels time to end the session.

Remove the stones beginning at the crown and removing the grounding stones last. Then, use a Selenite wand at the very end to clear and smooth the auric field.

Releasing Cellular Memory Technique

This technique is to assist your client in discovering their own blocked and hidden memories. It is vitally important that you do not interfere with the client's process by instilling your own will, advice, opinion or counseling into the session. Your responsibility is to hold a safe environment for your client to explore and process what arises from the cellular memory.

It is very tempting to think that we know more about the client's life then the client does but you must sit with integrity and allow them to use this time for self-exploration without interfering in the process. I cannot stress this enough! Unless you are a certified counselor, do not counsel! Simply follow the steps and be a safe heart for them during the process.

You may ask two questions during the session:

- What are you feeling?

- Where are you feeling this in your body?

Simply allow them to feel. If the client wants to talk, allow them the space to express themselves. This is a time for your client to be heard, not for you to instill your self-proclaimed wisdom on them.

If this sounds like a harsh guideline, let me explain that you are responsible for any advice or counseling that you give and your reputation as a healing practitioner is on the line. It's much better to be cautious here and honor that your client is wise and has all the answers they need inside of themselves. This layout will assist them in unlocking those answers.

In addition to the stones, you will need a laser wand, extra Azurite and two tumbled Obsidian stones.

Layout:

Next to Ankles: Lingams – For grounding and stability

In between legs: Black Tourmaline – For grounding and alignment

Thighs: Galena – Grounding and transformation

Second Chakra: Azurite – Unlock frozen memories

Third Chakra: Amber – Draw out memories; transmute negativity

Fourth Chakra: Malachite – Draw out emotional blocks

Fifth Chakra: Chrysocolla – Allows truth and inner wisdom to surface

Sixth Chakra: Azurite – Brings up innate knowledge

Seventh Chakra: Laser wand pointed towards crown – opens crown

Hands: Petrified Wood – Unlocking the past

Before you begin, have a chat with your client to review area(s) of discomfort on the physical body or the emotional discomfort she/he is experiencing. Connect to each other by holding hands repeating the Light Invocation three times: I invoke the Light of the Christ within. I am a clear and perfect channel. Light is my guide.

Have your client get on the table. Clear the stones and place them on the body starting at the ankles and ending at the crown chakra.

Place additional pieces of azurite directly on the area(s) of discomfort with the blue side facing downward to the body. Lay your hands-on top of that piece of Azurite and sit quietly as the energy permeates into the cellular structure. Instruct your client to concentrate on that area taking in slow, deep breaths.

After about five minutes, draw counterclockwise circles around that piece of Azurite with your laser wand. Draw the energy out and upward, flicking it upward and allowing the Universe to transmute the energy. Do this twelve times.

Once again, place your hands-on top of the azurite and ask your client to relay how they are feeling. Ask her/him if they have any memories coming up. Hold space for them by just allowing them to talk. Do not counsel or direct their conversation. Simply let them lead the healing.

If the client doesn't experience anything, replace the petrified wood in their hands with black obsidian. Once again draw counterclockwise with the Laser crystal around the piece of Azurite. Allow the azurite to do the work.

At intervals, ask your client how they are feeling emotionally. Keep it simple: mad, sad, glad, hurt, scared or ashamed and also how they physically feel. Get a sense of any resistance they may be feeling doing this work. Never push them to respond or lead them to a response that you feel they should have. Unless you are a certified therapist, you are not qualified to give advice. Remember, this is a process and everyone processes at a different rate or, in some cases, not at all. Respect your client's process.

You may feel like doing some form of hands-on energy work during this process in order to relax your client and open the energy centers. Continue to go back to the area with the Azurite and to periodically check in with your client.

If your client becomes emotional, allow them the space to do so. Do not stop an emotional outburst unless you or the client are being physically harmed. Simply hold the space for your client to feel safe and secure enough to process their emotions.

At the end of the session, use your laser wand to draw clockwise around the area of the Azurite to close the circle. Once again, place your hands on the Azurite for a few minutes for closure. Then, remove the stones beginning at their crown chakra and finishing at the ankles. Clear them.

Allow your client to lie on the table until she/he feels ready to sit up. Rub their back, their arms and their legs to bring them back into their body. Check their eyes to make sure they are fully present and ready to stand up. Give them a glass of water, or a cracker or cookie, just to make certain that they are grounded and centered.

Advise your client to journal their experience and, if necessary, repeat this healing technique until they feel they have fully removed the cellular blockages from this particular circumstance. You may want to follow up in a day or so with a phone call to ensure that they are all right. Again, unless you are a certified therapist, you are not qualified to give advice or counsel. Your part in this is to hold space for your client to feel and express themselves.

I highly suggest that my clients find a qualified therapist to follow up with in order to process their feelings and discoveries. I keep a list of therapists in my healing room to give out as references.

<u>Releasing Fear Healing Technique</u>

Everyone has fear – if you are a human being, you have fear. Fear is the emotion that holds us back the most from actualizing who we truly are. There are only two natural fears – the fear of falling and the fear of sudden, loud noises – the rest have been taught to us by our families, religions, friends, the media, teachers – you name it, it's all over the place. Fear prevents us from doing the things we truly want to do or become who we truly know we can be.   A wonderful friend of mine used to ask me, "What would you do if you had no fear?" This question really made me think and feel to the point where I knew I had to do something to alleviate and overcome my fears.

This layout and healing are designed to assist in safely bringing our fears to the forefront so that we can become aware of them, understand their genesis in our lives and question the validity of their power over us. It is through awareness and courage that we can conquer the anxiety, shyness, panic, shame and lack of self-confidence that fear presents to us.

Have your client bring a notebook and pen to this session so that they can journal afterward what arises during the session. This is designed to be gentle and non-invasive allowing for a safe space for them to heal.

As with any healing session, unless you are a certified therapist, it is not your job to counsel anyone during or after the healing. You are there to be the container for your client and respect their process with gratitude and humility.

In addition to the chakra stones, you will need two Citrine points.

Layout:

Between the Ankles – Lingam

In between legs – Black Tourmaline

Thighs – Petrified Wood

Second chakra – Moonstone

Third chakra – Citrine Cluster points facing downward

Fourth chakra – Rose Quartz

Fifth chakra – Turquoise

Sixth chakra – Ametrine

Seventh chakra – Danburite

Hands – Citrine

Once your client has settled comfortably on the table, begin by holding the ankles and bring your client's energy and attention into their root chakra. Hold this position until you feel their energy coming down to meet your hands.

Place your Citrine points in your hands, with the left-hand crystal's termination point facing the wrist and the right-hand crystal's termination point facing the fingertips.

Next, ground and center yourself. When you are ready say the Light Invocation three times: *I invoke the light of Universal Energy within. I am a clear and perfect channel. Light is my guide.*

Next, place the left-hand crystal flush on the bottom of the left foot and the right-hand crystal flush on the bottom of the right foot. This is the nervous system balancing.

Next, say the Light Invocation to activate a five-minute cycle and hold the crystals steady for the duration of the cycle. After five minutes, remove the crystals from the bottoms of the feet and go to the hip area. Find the indented area right below the hip bone on each side of the hips and place one crystal point facing in on one hip and one crystal point facing out at the other. Both terminations should be going in the same direction. This is the circulatory balancing.

Repeat the Light Invocation three times to activate the five-minute cycle. After five minutes, slowly remove the crystals from the hips.

Next move to the top of the client's head. Place the left-handed point facing the wrist and the right-handed crystal facing the fingertips. Gently place the crystals on either side of the head near the temples so as not to cause discomfort. This is the brain balancing.

Repeat the Light Invocation three times to activate the five-minute cycle. When you are finished, slowly remove the crystals from the sides of the head and clear them by saying the Light Invocation three times.

Next, move back to the client's feet and hold one Citrine point on the bottom of one foot and the other under the knee. Pause until you feel it's time to move. Then, still holding the Citrine points, hold one Citrine on the top of the hip joint and the other underneath the knee. Again, hold this position for as long as you feel is needed. Repeat both positions on the client's other side, making sure to pause as needed.

Move to the client's hips and hold one Citrine on each hip with the points facing in towards the body. Run energy between the points. Then, use a counter-clockwise circular motion to open the second chakra with the Citrine point and draw out negativity from the area. Release it either into the ground or out of the auric field. When you feel that the area is clear, draw clockwise around the area and hold the Citrine on the area.

Move to third chakra and use the same counter-clock circular motion to open this chakra and draw out any negative energies. Release it and close the area by drawing clockwise around the area. Repeat with the fourth chakra.

Place the Citrine points on either side of the client's neck and hold for a few moments, then place the Citrine points gently on the sides of the head. When you feel that the head is calm and relaxed, remove the points and the layout stones from the body starting from the crown down to the ankles.

Clear the stones by repeating the Light Invocation three times: I invoke the light of Universal Energy within. I am a clear and perfect channel. Light is my guide.

To end the session, fluff the layers of the field with a Citrine point and gently rake the client's body starting at the arms and working your way down to the feet. Hold their ankles and allow them to feel their physicality before sitting up. Then, rub their arms, their back and legs until they are fully alert.

Give them their journal and allow them time to write their experience.

<u>Releasing the Need to Be Perfect</u>

This simple meditation is perfect for releasing that critical inner voice that demands perfection at all times. You will need an Obsidian sphere, and Azurite and Kunzite stones.

Begin by finding a quiet space to work and a journal. Take some time and write down an area in your life where you feel the need to be perfect. Next, gaze into an obsidian sphere until you 'see' how that is affecting your life. Journal all the ways that it is preventing you from actualizing who you truly are.

After you've finished journaling, lie down on a mat and set the Azurite on a place of your body where you feel the blockage of this. Give yourself time to truly feel into the emotions of this blockage and allow the Azurite to release the thoughts, events and reluctance to move forward.

When you have completed this part, take the azurite off and replace it with the Kunzite to fill the space with unconditional love and acceptance. Allow yourself the freedom to feel your self-excellence and self-approval.

When you're ready, journal what you have discovered, felt, released. Next, write down a course of personal action that you can take to shift any feelings of low self-esteem, guilt, pessimism, rigidity, obsessiveness, immobilization, procrastination, or lack of belief in yourself.

<u>Sinus Opening with Crystals</u>

This technique is designed to assist a release in the sinus cavities. It will bring relief from allergies, colds, sinusitis, stuffiness and grief. In addition to the chakra stones, you will need two small laser crystals.

Layout:

Below Feet at the heels – Striated Selenite Wands

In Between Legs – Black Tourmaline

Second chakra – Green Calcite

Third chakra – Malachite

Fourth chakra – Green Calcite

Fifth chakra – Blue Kyanite Blade

Next to the Nose – Small Blue Kyanite Blades

Sixth chakra – Blue Kyanite Blade

Seventh chakra – Green Calcite

Hands – Apache Tears

Begin by clearing the stones and placing them on the body beginning at the feet with the crown chakra stone last.

Place your fingertips on the occipital ridge under the head. Simultaneously run energy and massage the area until you sense that it is loosening and becoming relaxed. This will allow your client to have a sense of comfort and ease in order to allow the energy to flow evenly and freely.

Clear the laser crystals by saying the Light Invocation three times: I invoke the light of Universal Energy within. I am a clear and perfect channel. Light is my guide. Gently place the tips of the crystals pointing towards the temples for about 10 seconds. You do not want to do this for longer as it can cause headaches but a short period of time allows for the mind to clear.

Place the crystal points lightly at the sides of the crown of the nose. Do this until you feel a flow of energy in this area. The time will differ with each individual.

Move the crystal points so that they are lightly at the top of the jaw and direct energy into this area. You may want to tell your client to gently open their mouth to loosen the tension in the jaw.

Using one laser crystal, begin to lightly direct energy from about ¼ inch below the eye near the side of the nose and run the crystal point down the nose, underneath and around the cheekbone, down the jawline and to the shoulder area. This will help to release the tension in the face and open the sinus area. Repeat this several times until you feel the energy begin to flow.

Repeat on the other side, lightly directing energy from about ¼ inch below the eye near the side of the nose and run the crystal point down the nose, underneath and around the cheekbone, down the jawline and to the shoulder area.

Lightly place the tips of the crystals ½ inch from the base of the nose at the end of the cheek bones facing upwards. Hold until you feel an opening in the nasal passages.

Next, lightly place the tips of each laser crystal underneath the cheek bones pointing up towards the eyes. Hold them here until you feel the tension release in the upper teeth.

Put the crystals aside and place your fingertips lightly on the top of the eyebrows and run energy down the face.

Place your fingertips beneath the eyes and stroke the face moving your fingers down towards the neck. Do this for several minutes while the sinuses have an opportunity to open and drain.

End the session by placing your fingertips back on the occipital ridge and gently massage the area. Remove the layout starting at the crown chakra and ending at the feet. Gently rake the body with your fingertips starting on the face and moving down the body to the feet.

Hold the ankles until the you feel their energy come down to your hands. When they arise, rub their arms, back and legs until they are fully present.

<u>Vertebral Healing</u>

This is not a traditional layout. You will need Smoky Quartz, Calcite, Fluorite, Selenite, Howlite and two Quartz healing wands.

Begin with client lying face up. Place your hands on the back of the client's neck. Begin at the upper thoracic vertebrae and work your way up to the base of the skull to get a feel for the tone of the muscles in the area.

Using the pads of your fingers, gently soften the muscles on each side of the vertebrae, one at a time starting at the base of the neck and working up to the base of the skull. Then, with your fingertips, clear out the area around the rim of the base of the skull just above the top vertebrae. Follow the rim of the skull all the way up to the back of the ears. This opens up the energy flow to the spine.

Gently tilt the head front to back, rotate the head from side to side and stretch it forward to check the range of motion. Place your fingertips off to the side of each vertebrae to give each vertebra independent motion. Take some time and send energy from your fingertips to each vertebra going up the neck.

Next, have the client turn face lie on their stomach with their head in a face cradle. On one side of the spine starting at the lower back and going up, place: Smoky Quartz, Calcite, Fluorite, Selenite and Howlite. Using thumbs and fingertips placed between the vertebrae on each side of the spine, micro-massage to free up the vertebrae.

Next, gently soften the long muscles running parallel to the spine with the palms of your hands. Then, place your hands on the sacrum and gently rock the pelvis noting the tone of the muscles and freedom of motion in the sacrum. It should feel like it's floating.

Feel along the iliosacral junction on each side of the sacrum and, with the fingertips, soften the muscles to free up the area.

Using a Quartz wand in each hand, send a line of light from the base of the spine up the spinal column with one of the points and hold the other crystal with the point facing down from the base of the brain stem to clear and balance the spine. Then check to see if the energy runs freely from the sacrum to the base of the skull by placing one hand on the base of the neck and one hand on the sacrum. If not, repeat the wand procedure.

Run crystal energy with the lower crystal point at the sacrum pointing up the spine while at the same time using the other crystal to run energy into each vertebra starting at the neck and working down the spine.

Remove the stones and place one hand on the back of the neck and the other on the lower back. Run energy from your hands into the back and then gently rock the client back and forth for a minute.

Have your client turn over and then hold their ankles until you feel that they are meeting your energy at the feet. When they arise, rub their arms, back and legs until they are fully present.

Chapter Thirteen

Everyone Needs a Go-To Reference

This chapter contains groupings of stones for various needs that people have. These are the most commonly requested lists from customers and students and give easy to understand explanations for each stone in order to keep it simple (Spirit)!

In our classes I give these lists to my students and allow them to intuitively choose from them to do self-healing and individual layouts. Our energy systems know exactly what they need and with these alphabetized reference lists, you can quickly choose the preferred stones required by your spirit.

Much of our inner healing is a matter of listening with our senses to what our body is asking us for. I encourage everyone to spend several minutes a day checking in with your energy system in order to become acquainted with how you feel physically, mentally, emotionally and spiritually.

When I first began doing this work, I did this simple exercise every morning when I woke up. I would close my eyes and put my hands on each chakra beginning at the root and ask, "How are you feeling today and what do you need from me?" Then I would write that down and proceed to the second chakra and repeat that until I was finished at the crown. I did my best each day to honor what each center was asking from me and, in that fashion, I learned how to tune in to my feelings and my senses.

Remember that healing is feeling and so much of this work is a repetition to learn how to feel. We spend a great deal of our lives ignoring our feelings and ignoring the inner voices that want to be heard. You will do yourself a great service if you spend even fifteen to twenty minutes a day practicing listening and feeling. Unfortunately, these are not two of the skills that are taught to us when we are young. Can you imagine how useful it would have been if our parents and teachers had the wisdom, time and patience to teach us these very basic life skills? But, it's never too late to start and now is a great time.

Use these lists as references for when your bodies, minds and spirits call to you for assistance. Be still and listen!

Stones for Calming the Mind

Amazonite	Balances female and male energies. Reminds us to not take ourself too seriously. Soothes the nervous system.
Apophyllite	Helps us to aspire to a state of perfection, of truth and Universal Love. Provides for clarity of thought and aligns all chakras to its energy.
Azurite	Helpful in remembering past lives, memories and to recall important information for healing purposes. Assists in developing psychic abilities.
Black Kyanite	Helps assimilate scattered root chakra energy in order to bring a person into balance and harmony.
Blue Kyanite	Aids the communication between ourself and Spirit for clear channeling.
Black Onyx	Draws out memories from our root chakra to guide us in emotional and spiritual healing. Assists in dealing with grief and anxiety.
Chiastolite	Grounds and centers in order to access spiritual energy throughout the chakra system. Helps us to be practical while at the same time becoming aware of our inner spiritual life.
Copper	Brings a steady and balancing flow of energy throughout our body while aligning our chakras to all levels of the field. Energizing and dynamic.
Danburite	Brings joyful energy through the crown chakra down into the heart. Opens our heart to the purity of their true essence.
Fluorite	Best for mental assimilation and concentration helping to clear scattered thought patterns. Great for students, teachers, computer programmers and other occupations requiring astute thinking.
Hematite	Very good for grounding, concentration, memory and staying connected with our bodies.

Herkimer	Great for inspiring and remembering dreams, assisting in clairvoyance and clairaudience. Helps us to release tension, stress and toxins.
Howlite	Promotes peacefulness and calm helping to alleviate stress and anxiety. Grounds and balances our sense of spirit to encourage living a life of honesty and harmony.
Jade	Assists in dreaming and solving life's uncertainties through the dream state. Aids in bringing our dreams into reality and manifesting what is for the highest good.
Jet	Helps alleviate fear, anxiety and money issues associated with lower back pain. Aligns our root chakra with the rest of our chakra system.
Kunzite	Assists in exploring the heart at the 'you' level by helping to find out what is preventing us from loving ourselves. Works with self-responsibility, self-reliance and self-sufficiency.
Lapis Lazuli	Used for mental and spiritual clarity. Helps in breaking down karmic patterns allowing for moving ahead on our spiritual path.
Lepidolite	The lithium base in Lepidolite helps to calm anxiety, bring a sense of peace and soothing our nervous system.
Malachite	Stimulates cellular memory to unlock stagnant feelings and emotional patterns in order to allow a more positive consciousness to enter.
Mochi Marbles	Balances male and female energies in order to align our chakras and keep our equilibrium. Excellent for removing energy blockages.
Moonstone	Assists in balancing moods and cycles of the body. Brings a sense of peace, calm and well-being.

Petrified Wood	Provides strength and grounding while allowing for transformation to occur within the cellular level of our body. Connects with all time and space.
Pietersite	Opens our third eye chakra to expand our thoughts in order make all things possible. Helps us to go beyond the ordinary, leaving behind black and white thinking.
Pyrite	Good for deflecting negativity. Aids in memory recall.
Quartz Crystal	Purifies, balances, restructures, regenerates, harmonizes, energizes, amplifies, releases blockages and connects and balances our chakras.
Selenite	Lifts us into a fine meditative state. Assists in developing telepathic communication skills and psychic abilities. Connects our meridians.
Star of the Sea	Opens and expands our chakras, bringing a calming effect. Connects us to our spiritual gifts and aids in peaceful sleep and pleasant dreams.
Sugilite	Connects our sixth chakra to the root chakra allowing for the Kundalini to flow. Opens us up to our inner calling and a fresh connection to the soul. Aids in eliminating hostility and for feeling freedom in life.
Zebra Skin Agate	Aligns our crown chakra to our root chakra in order to balance and ground spiritual energy throughout the body. Promotes determination and discipline in order to move through layers of disillusionment.

Stones for Cellular Healing

Azurite	Aids in revealing the reason(s) we continue to hold onto chronic pain and the genesis of our fears. While cleansing and strengthening the emotional body, it assists the cells in releasing old belief systems and conditionings.
Elestials	Brings forward information and enlightenment to assist in breaking the code of blocked cellular memory. Aligns with our root chakra ground and center us. Works on the nodal cord area to unlock the past and give clarity as to the patterns we have lived with.
Galena	Helps overcome the fear that prevents us from continuing our spiritual journey. Assists in regaining our personal power and strengthens our resolve to know who we truly are. Works to counter the ill effects of radiation and electromagnetic fields.
Labradorite	Provides intuitive wisdom needed dispel illusion to the root cause of an issue. Aids in releasing negative thoughts and beliefs held in the cellular structure. Assists in deflecting negativity from our auric field.
Laser Wands	Acts as a direct form of energy, permeating the physical body and helping to redistribute and align cells in a healthy pattern. Assists in releasing hidden memory, past life patterns, and injuries – both emotional and physical – in order to gain awareness and move forward with clarity and a renewed sense of spirit.
Petrified Wood	Helps with unlocking past life experiences which so often are the genesis of our blocked cellular memory. A grounding stone. Provides an emotional safety net and courage when delving into the realms of the past.

Stones for Emotions

Anger

Blue Lace Agate	Promotes calm when speaking. Helps us to think before we speak. Assists in working through anger issues.
Blue Calcite	Expands our throat chakra and brings a calm presence to our speech. Promotes a gentle and peaceful demeanor.
Green Calcite	Softens the heart energy anywhere on our body promoting peace and tranquility.
Chrysoprase	Promotes calming of the heart and both acceptance of self and others. Aids in forgiveness, compassion and empathy. Helps to lower high blood pressure.

Sadness

Apache Tears	Assists in seeing through the veils our grief in order to help bring comfort and release from suffering.
Black Onyx	Draws out memories from our root chakra to guide in emotional and spiritual healing. Assists in dealing with grief and anxiety.
Rose Quartz	Helps in overcoming heartache and emotional turmoil by helping us to release sadness. Assists in attracting new love into our life by helping us to understand that love is deserved by everyone.

Joy

Amazonite	Balances our female and male energies. Helps us to not take ourself too seriously. Soothes the nervous system.
Angelite	Connects us to our guides and angels with a very refined vibration, helping to find answers about our gifts and talents. Opens our telepathic channels.
Apophyllite	Helps us to aspire to a state of perfection, of truth and Universal Love. Provides for clarity of thought and aligns all chakras to its energy.
Danburite	Brings joyful energy through our crown chakra down into our heart. Opens our heart to the purity of our true essence.
Peacock Ore	Opens and expands our auric field, bringing forth lightness and joy. Gently guides us to seek the lightness of life and release our shadow.
Rhodochrosite	Connects our heart chakra with our crown chakra, allowing Universal love to enter. Works with connecting our dualities to help us understanding them. Helps balance our feelings and promotes joy.
Spirit Quartz	Transforms stagnant thought patterns into positive, joyful feelings, freeing us from the chains of the past. Connects us to guides and angels while in the meditative state.
Topaz	Can be used to help gain an enlightened state. Softens the human will and allows our Soul's will to become prevalent. Brings joyful energy.

Hurt

Celestite	Brings in heavenly perceptions from the spiritual realm and assists in the communication of the information. Helps to clarify complex concepts in order to aid in changing outmoded belief systems.
Hiddenite	Goes deep into the heart to bring forth veiled wounds. Helps us understand the need to heal our wounds in order to bring joy and love into our life.
Howlite	Promotes peacefulness and calm, helping to alleviate stress and anxiety. Grounds and balances our sense of spirit. Encourages us to live a life of honesty and harmony.
Morganite	Goes to the depth of the heart in order to 'show' us that love that is available if we choose to work on our issues. Makes possible the growth necessary to live a life free of judgement.
Star of the Sea	Opens and expands our chakras, bringing a calming feeling to our emotions. Connects us to our spiritual gifts. Aids in peaceful sleep and pleasant dreams.
Tourmaline Green	Expands our heart chakra and directs the heart energy throughout our chakra system. Assists in helping us to believe in ourself, leaving behind childhood conditioning and etched thought patterns.

Fear

Amethyst	Opens us to our own inner knowing and connects us to spiritual nature. Helps us to attain serene state. Supports meditation and peaceful sleep. Assists in breaking addictions.
Ametrine	Clears negativity and fear to allow us to go beyond our perception of what is possible. Aids in astral travel so that we can see things from a different perspective.
Apatite	Provides us the courage to release old patterns and destructive habits. Brings freedom from attachment and helps us to move forward into healthier living.
Aquamarine	Known as the "Stone of Courage and Truth." Allows for clarity of thought. Helps us to understand the truths of the Universe.
Azurite	Helpful in remembering our past lives, memories, and to recall important information for healing purposes. Assists in developing our psychic abilities.
Charoite	Thrusts us forward through life's lessons. Helps us to experience each lesson on a 'gut' level in order to integrate the experience, learn from it and move on. Challenges us to make real and lasting change.
Chrysocolla	Assists us to express ourselves. Provides the confidence we need to speak freely in front of groups, and helps us to know when to be quiet. Promotes endurance in difficult situations.
Citrine	"Fear breaker" helps us to see the core of our fear in order to grow past it. Good for manifestation and abundance.
Leopardskin Jasper	Breaks up our resistance to change, allowing for a more fluid existence. Instills courage and determination to move forward in our own endeavors.
Jet	Helps to alleviate fear, anxiety and money issues. Aligns our root chakra with the rest of the chakra system.

Larimar	Helps unchain our fears to allow for a sense of true freedom and fulfillment. Provides an opportunity to relax and flow with life.
Orange Calcite	Gently prods us to exercise our own ambitions while helping alleviate the fear surrounding the change. Expansive in a non-assuming way.

Shame

Amber	Draws out negativity and transmutes it into positive energy. Helps us develop a feeling of calmness, self-confidence and unconditional love.
Bronzite	Promotes a state of being non-judgmental, giving us sufficient confidence to love ourselves in order to hold others in a place of compassion.
Carnelian	Restores our motivation and encourages us to trust ourselves and our instincts. Helps us to promote our talents and skills.
Moonstone	Calms our emotions and gently alleviates emotional triggers. Supports emotional intelligence to help us identify and dissolve outdated emotional patterns.
Opal	Helps us to understand our true nature, alleviating feelings of being unworthy. Reduces inhibitions and allows for the fulfillment of dreams.
Picture Jasper	Grounds our creativity so that we can complete projects and tasks in an enjoyable way. Good for bringing forward the pain of buried emotions in order to deal with the root cause.
Ruby	Enhances our sexual relationships. Helps us express anger in a healthy way and to use our creativity to move forward in this life.

All

Azurite — Helpful in remembering our past lives, memories, and to recall important information for healing purposes. Assists in developing psychic abilities.

Black Obsidian — Delves into our shadow side to assist us in seeing that part of ourselves. Helps with breaking addictions.

Kunzite — Assists in exploring the heart at the 'you' level by helping us to find out what is preventing us from loving ourselves. Helps us approach life with self-responsibility, self-reliance and self-sufficiency.

Lepidolite — Natural lithium content assists in calming anxiety and working with depression. Stimulates the feeling of self-love and self-acceptance.

Malachite — Stimulates cellular memory to unlock stagnant feelings and emotional patterns in order to allow a more positive consciousness to enter.

Ruby — Encourages us to have a passion for life. Helps us express anger in a healthy way and to use our creativity to move forward in this life.

Grounding Stones

Apache Tears	Assists us to see through the veils of our grief to help bring us comfort and release from suffering. Provides grounding after working with higher frequency stones.
Black Kyanite	Helps assimilate our scattered root chakra energy in order to bring us into balance and harmony. Can clear blocked energy in all chakras. Helps to repair holes and tears in the levels of the field.
Black Obsidian	Helps us ground and center for self-actualization. Aids in shielding us from negative energies. Known as the "Shadow Stone" as it assists us in looking at our shadow side.
Black Onyx	Draws out hidden memories for emotional and spiritual healing. Assist with grief and anxiety. Also helps provide stamina as it prevents the draining of our emotional and physical energy.
Black Tourmaline	Called "Roto Rooter" as it helps to open up and align all of our chakras. Great stone for protecting our aura from outside negativity as well as being one of the premier stones for grounding.
Boji Stones	Balances our male and female energies in order to align our chakras and keep our equilibrium. Excellent for removing energy blockages caused by emotional problems. Assist in bringing excess nervous energy down to the feet and into the earth.
Chiastolite	Supports us to grounds and center so that we can access spiritual energy throughout our chakra system. Assists us to be practical while becoming aware of our inner spiritual life.
Copper	Soothes our nervous system. Brings a steady and balancing flow of energy to assist with aligning our chakras to all levels of our auric field. Energizing and dynamic.

Dravite	Helps us to let go of self-doubt. Aligns our chakras to give us a sense of inner cooperation. Helps to bring higher vibrations down through our chakra system to ground and center. Aids in bringing more stamina to our physicality.
Hematite	Provides us with the grounding we need to stay in the moment. Assists with memory, concentration, and staying connected with our bodies.
Jet	Draws out issues of fear from our root chakra. Adds in alleviating anxiety and to calm our nervous system. Draws out negativity and protects us from outside influences.
Lingam	Provides a feeling of balances and grounding. Instills sacred attitude in all aspects of our lives. Brings the male and female aspects together. Assists in the rising of the Kundalini. Helps us to connect to the Divine.
Nuummite	Patches tears in our aura. Provides protection from negative forces. Good for soul retrieval work as it integrates pieces which have been separated from ourself. Supports mental and psychic healing.
Petrified Wood	Assists in grounding, past life remembrance, and breaking our karmic patterns. Stabilizes our emotions and calms survival-based fears. A foundational stone; helps establish new goals and change course in our lives.
Pyrite	Good for deflecting negativity from our aura. Assists in memory recall. Known as the "Traveler's Stone" as it is said to protect those who travel.
Smoky Quartz	A grounding stone that supports releasing our anxiety and sadness without falling apart. Naturally radiated; supports recovery from cancer treatment.
Zebra Skin Agate	Aligns our crown chakra to our root chakra to balance and ground our spiritual energy. Promotes determination and discipline in order to accomplish tasks. Provides fortitude to live our life as we wish.

<u>Heart Stones</u>

Aventurine	Energy from this stone goes where it is needed. Promotes feelings of joy, of daydreams coming true and of the possibilities of all things.
Chrysoprase	Promotes calming of the heart and acceptance of both ourselves and others. Aids in forgiveness, compassion and empathy. Helps to lower high blood pressure.
Dioptase	Gives us the energy and initiative to separate the 'wheat from the chafe' in order to have confidence and faith in living life the way we choose.
Emerald	Works with our heart to connect to all of our chakras. A good relationship stone that promotes fidelity and loyalty in relationship.
Green Calcite	Softens our heart energy when placed anywhere on our body. Promotes feelings of peace and tranquility. Helps to release that which no longer serves our highest good.
Green Tourmaline	Expands our heart chakra and directs this heart energy throughout our chakra system. Helps us to believe in ourselves, leaving behind childhood conditioning and etched thought patterns.
Hiddenite	Goes deep into our heart to bring forth veiled wounds for healing. Helps us to truly understand our need to heal emotional wounds in order to bring joy and love into our lives.
Jade	Supports insightful dreaming and solving our life's uncertainties through the dream state. Aids in bringing our dreams into reality and manifesting what is for the highest good.
Kunzite	Awakens our heart chakra to allow unconditional self-love. Encourages self-expression and repairs lost trust. It can help us clear emotional debris and recapture our lost innocence.

Morganite	Goes to the depth of our heart in order to 'show' us the love that is available if we choose to work on our own issues. Provides a path needed to live a life free of self-judgement.
Pink Quartz	Supports a gently search for secrets that we have hidden secrets from ourselves in order to release blocked trauma. Nurtures self-love, compassion and trust. Not to be confused with Rose Quartz.
Pink Tourmaline	Lithium in this stone provides a calming effect that promotes joy and light. A mood shifter; assists lifting our spirit and connecting our heart chakra to our crown and bringing in a clearer state of mind.
Rhodochrosite	Connects our heart chakra with our crown chakra, allowing Universal love to enter. Works to connect dualities and helps us to understand them. Supports our ability to balance our feelings and promotes joy.
Rhodonite	Connects our heart chakra with our root chakra to help ground our heart energies. Aids with relationship communication and understanding the nuances within our relationships.
Rose Quartz	Helps in overcoming heartache and emotional turmoil by helping us to release sadness. Helps us to attract new love into our life by helping us to understand that love is deserved by everyone.
Seraphinite	Supports us to become aligned to the goodness of the earth in order to respect all living things. Connects our chakra system to the spiritual level of the auric field.
Unakite	This double heart chakra stone helps to align and balance our heart. It assists us to appreciate who we are through self-acceptance and self-love.

Stones for Impeccability

Amber	Draws out negativity and transmutes it into positive energy. Helps us to develop self-confidence. Gives us a stronger sense of our true self to help us to live from a place of truth and self-compassion.
Amethyst	Purifies our aura of any negative energy or attachments. Creates a protective shield, allowing use to remain centered while being open for spiritual direction. Calms angry temperaments. Assists in curbing bad habits.
Ametrine	Supports letting go and releasing fear. Aids in meditation, boosts psychic abilities, relieves tension, disperses negativity and helps to eliminate prejudice. Assists in releasing negative memories. A combination of Amethyst and Citrine.
Apophyllite	Aids meditation and connection to the spiritual world. Helps us to see the truth and act on it. Assists in self-reflection in order to correct undesirable behavior. Helps clairvoyance and seeing into the future.
Aquamarine	Allows for clarity of thought. Helps overcome the fear of speaking, and is an excellent stone for teachers and presenters of all types. Supports speaking clearly and without anger in difficult situations.
Black Obsidian	Delves into our 'shadow' side to help us to truly see that part of ourselves. Assists us to examine unresolved issues. Support our work on ancestral and family lines.
Blue Lace Agate	Helps us to speak without anger. Assists in clearing communication. Inspires loyalty and trustworthiness.
Bronzite	Support our need to be of service and assistance to the world. Provides a clear foundation to explore our chosen lifepath. Promotes our ability to be non-judgmental. Gives courage to follow our hearts.
Charoite	Encourages us to integrate our life experiences, learn from them, and to move on. Assists in releasing fear and negativity. Aligns our heart with our intellect.

Chevron Amethyst	Enhances peace of mind, relaxation, courage and inner strength. Strong, focused energy for dissipating and repelling negativity. Combines the strengthening qualities of Quartz with the stress-relieving qualities of Amethyst.
Citrine	Works with fear and self-esteem issues to break the stories of our past. Allows us to move forward with clarity and truth. Gives us the courage to always live our lives with impeccability.
Emeralds	Brings feelings of love, romance and joy. Supports truthfulness, mental clarity and perception. Valuable to those seeking trust.
Green Calcite	Releases limiting beliefs brought on by fear. Helps us to go through transitions more gracefully.
Hiddenite	Helps us to relieve loss, particularly of love and money. Calming, helps engender compassion for others. Brings trust to relationships, especially with ourself.
Howlite	Spurs us into action to attain our goals. Aids in memory. Connects us to spiritual guidance and purity by connecting our crown chakra to our root chakra.
K-2	Supports moving forward and staying on task. Breaks down resistance between our ego and our spiritual nature. Connects our sacral chakra to our solar plexus chakra. This stone is a combination of Granite and Azurite.
Kunzite	A powerful emotional healer. Helps us let go of the fears and sorrows of our past and to be receptive to the opportunities life has to offer. Encourages us to be open to unconditional and abundant love.
Lapis Lazuli	A "Stone of Truth." Encourages honesty in spoken and written word. Supports mental and spiritual clarity. Helps us to break down karmic patterns in order to move forward in life. Excellent for enhancing memory.

Lepidolite | Assists us to calm anxiety and to work through depression. Stimulates the feeling of self-love and self-acceptance. Awakens a spiritual sense of love for ourselves and others due to natural lithium content in the stone.

Malachite | Encourages change and emotional risk-taking. Assists us in expressing our feelings. Supports breaking unwanted ties and outdated patterns. Sometimes referred to as the "Stone of Transformation."

Morganite | Encourages equality in all relationships. Rekindles compassion, empathy, self-control, patience. Connects our heart to Universal love and compassion. Called the "Courage Stone of the Heart" as it supports living a life of unconditional love.

Orange Calcite | Serves as a catalyst for the release of past trauma that is holding us back. Draws out old energy patterns to increase our motivation and drive. Draws out personal negativity, allowing optimism and joy to enter.

Pietersite | Enhances courage, tenacity, and the ability to create what we want. Works to release deep emotional blocks in a calm manner. Supports our ability to experience visions, precognition, working with angels, interdimensional travel.

Ruby | Promotes a courageous attitude and self-confidence. Supports increased concentration, a clear mind and personal motivation. Helps us to share loving energy despite past traumas. Encourages positivity.

Sugilite | Allows us to recognize and release sorrow, frustration, past angers and fear. Helps us internalize that living our own truth is both healing and empowering. Shines the light of love into the darkest moments of our lives. Known as the "Love Stone."

Tiger Eye | Teaches balance by helping us to understand the unity behind apparent opposite views. Supports the integration of spiritual aspects of our lives. Brings a practical and compassionate reasoning to our choices.

Stones for Physical Healing

Amethyst	Helps us to achieve a serene state as it works with us to reduce stress and improve circulation. Assists in breaking addictions. Balances our pineal and pituitary glands.
Apache Tears	Assists in calming muscle spasms. Enhances our immune system as it helps release sadness from the heart.
Apophyllite	Helpful in treating allergies and asthma. Works to reduce anxiety, fear response and stress-related headaches. Opens our pineal gland.
Aquamarine	Reduces throat inflammation, swollen glands and helps reduce allergic reactions, such as hay fever. Balances our larynx to ease communication.
Azurite	Soothes migraine headaches. Helpful for arthritis and joint pain. Balances our pineal and pituitary glands.
Black Tourmaline	Aligns our organs by stimulating our reflex points on our feet, ankles, lower back, and spine. Works to strengthen our immune system.
Bloodstone	Aids in clearing blood infections, bladder problems and cleansing the liver and kidneys. An excellent blood cleanser; stimulates our lymphatic system to heal inflammation.
Blue Kyanite	Provides natural pain relief. Helps to clear the sinus area and our throat due to allergies or infection. Assists in healing infections and to lower blood pressure.
Carnelian	Gently opening up our sexual centers. Aids in digestion and also has been known to alleviate lower back pain.
Chlorite Quartz	Aids in cleansing the entire energy system of the body. Good for purification of our entire organ system. Promotes manifestation by clearing out unwanted negative thoughts that bring a mentality of lack.

Chrysocolla — Helps to reduce arthritis and other bone-related disease. Works to elevate deep muscle cramps by strengthen our muscles. Draws out inflammation of the lungs.

Chrysoprase — Helps to lower high blood pressure. Balances our hormones. Assists in easing the strain of pregnancies and labor.

Citrine — Helps to calm our stomach in difficult situations. Works to help rebalance chemical imbalances and detoxify our blood.

Emerald — Aids our recovery after an infectious disease by stimulating our immune system. Supports our heart, lungs, spine and our muscles.

Fluorite — Strengthens our bone tissue to help with arthritis and injuries. Supports healing ulcers and respiratory tract infections.

Garnet — Stimulates our metabolism. Boosts our immune system and reduce toxins in the body. Acts as a cleansing agent for the colon.

Green Calcite — Assist with bacterial infections and works with our thymus to boost our autoimmune response. It calms our body's adrenal response.

Hematite — Supports our kidneys and helps regenerate tissues. Helps with the absorption of iron. Assist in aligning the spine and with fractures.

Jade — Aids our body's filtration and elimination organs. Excellent for treating kidney problems and adrenal glands.

Kunzite — Works to strengthen both the heart and our circulatory system. Calms nerve endings and joint pain. Stimulates our immune system.

Lapis Lazuli — Boosts our auto-immune response. Aids in regulating the thyroid and in lowering blood pressure.

Lepidolite	Natural lithium content assists in calming anxiety and works with depression. Assists in balancing our adrenal glands and kidneys.
Lingam	Assists with fertility issues and prostate health by restoring balance to our whole body.
Malachite	Boosts our immune system and stimulates our liver to release toxins from our body. Great for sprains, strains, arthritis pain, carpal tunnel, tendonitis and swelling.
Moonstone	Supports the digestive system and eliminates toxins from the body. Alleviates cramping due to menstrual cycles and assists in the birthing process. Aids both male and female reproductive organs.
Pyrite	Aids the immune system in the treatment of our respiratory system. Helps reduce swelling and to lower fevers.
Quartz Crystal	Known as the "Master Healer" as it helps to stimulate our immune system. It enhances our energy flow to bring our bodies back into balance. This crystal has the closest vibration of any stone to that of the human body.
Red Jasper	Supports energetic balancing in all of our organs, including the digestive, circulatory and male and female reproductive organs.
Rose Quartz	Beneficial in fertility and the birthing process. Strengthens our physical heart and supports our circulatory system.
Ruby	Enhances sexual relationships. Supports male and female reproductive organs, gall bladder and liver.
Seraphinite	Helpful in cleansing organs and refining our body's energy system. Supports healing our physical nerves and brain cells.
Sodalite	Cleanses our lymphatic system and provides stability and support for our throat, vocal cords and larynx. Helps balance the thyroid.

Star of the Sea   Supports deep, peaceful sleep and pleasant dreams. Assists deep healing on the cellular level. Supports our stomach, pancreas, and spleen.

Sugilite   Brings the left and right sides of our brain into balance. Relieves emotional disturbances, relieve insomnia and to channel healing energies where we need it. Balances the pineal and pituitary glands.

Tiger Eye   Releases toxins in our bodies, works to alleviate pain and to cleanses the liver, stomach and intestines.

Turquoise   Supports increased nutritional absorption. Believed to as an anti-inflammatory agent to soothe muscular cramps. Clears inflammation from the lungs.

Stones for Self-Esteem

Amber	Draws out negativity and transmutes it into positive energy. Helps us in developing calmness, self-confidence and unconditional love.
Amethyst	Gradually opens us to our own inner knowing and connects us to our spiritual nature. Helps in attaining serenity. Good for meditation and peaceful sleep. Assists in breaking addictions.
Ametrine	Clears negativity and fear to allow the openness necessary to go beyond our own perception of what is possible.
Apatite	Gives us the courage to release old patterns and the need for destructive habits. Brings freedom from attachment(s) and enables us to move forward to healthier living.
Aquamarine	Known as the "Stone of Courage and Truth." Allows for clarity of thought and helps us to understand the truths of the Universe.
Azurite	Helpful in remembering past lives, memories, and to recall important information for emotional healing. Assists in developing psychic abilities.
Bronzite	Promotes a state of being non-judgmental. Gives us that essential confidence to love ourselves in order to hold others in a place of compassion.
Charoite	Thrusts us forward through life's lessons so that we can experience each lesson at a 'gut' level. This helps us to integrate the experience, learn from it and move on. Challenges us to change.
Citrine	Known as the "Fear Breaker." Helps to get at the core of our fear in order to quiet it. Supports manifestation and abundance.
Danburite	Brings joyful energy through our crown chakra and into our heart. Opens our heart to the purity of our own true essence.

Garnet

Heightens our creativity and supports ability to use our unique talents to reach our lifelong ambitions. Commits us to our higher purpose.

Green Tourmaline

Expands our heart chakra and directs this energy throughout the entire chakra system. Assists in helping us to believe in ourself, leaving behind childhood conditioning and etched thought patterns.

Hematite

Very good for grounding, concentration, memory and staying connected with our bodies.

Howlite

Promotes a sense of peacefulness and calmness, helping to alleviate stress and anxiety. Grounds and balances our sense of spirit to encourage living a life of honesty and harmony.

Jade

Assists in solving life's uncertainties through the dream state. Aids in bringing our dreams into reality and manifesting what is for the highest good.

Leopard Skin Jasper

Breaks up our resistance to change, allowing for a more fluid existence. Helps instill courage and determination to move forward in our lives.

Picture Jasper

Grounds our creativity into completing projects and tasks in an enjoyable way. Supports bringing forward the pain of buried emotions in order to deal with the root cause.

Jet

Helps alleviate fear and anxiety by drawing out the negative energies in our aura. Supports our understanding what lesson needs to be learned from the experience.

Kunzite

Calming and protective. Connects us to self-love by helping us release energy blockages. Enhances our creativity, self-reliance and self-sufficiency.

Lapis Lazuli

Used for mental and spiritual clarity. Quickly releases stress. Helps us in breaking down karmic patterns, allowing us to move ahead on our spiritual path.

Lepidolite	Natural lithium content assists in calming anxiety to help us to work though depression. Stimulates the feeling of self-love and self-acceptance.
Malachite	Stimulates cellular memory to unlock stagnant feelings and emotional patterns in order to allow a more positive consciousness to enter.
Morganite	Goes deep into the depths of our heart in order to 'show' us the love that is available if we choose to work on our issues. Supports our growth to live a life free of self-judgement.
Obsidian	Forms a shield around us to protect from negativity. Stimulates our ability to clear our mind and helps to clear confusion. Helps to dissolve emotional blockages so we can heal.
Petrified Wood	Supports emotional strength and grounding. Helps us to be patient with ourselves and others, allowing for personal transformation to occur at its own pace.
Rose Quartz	Helps us to overcome heartache and emotional turmoil by aiding us to the release sadness. Assists in attracting new love into our life by helping us to realize that love is deserved by everyone.
Spirit Quartz	Transforms stagnant thought patterns into positive, joyful feelings to free ourselves from the chains of the past. Connects us to guides and angels while in the meditative state.
Sugilite	Connects our sixth chakra to our root chakra, allowing for the Kundalini to flow. This opens us up to our inner calling and provides a connection to our soul. Aids in eliminating hostility and for feeling freedom in life.
Tiger Eye	Guards against unwanted energies in our second chakra. Supports that 'gut' feeling when we are acting on ambitions and dreams. Helps build self-confidence and self-awareness.

Turquoise	Connects our throat to both the Earth and Spirit to provide both balance and courage. Brings things into alignment with Universal Law.

Stones for Stress and Anxiety

First Chakra

Apache Tears	Helps us to accept and to release grief and sorrow without feeling guilt.
Black Onyx	Gently draws issues out of our root chakra to alleviate trauma and anxiety.
Chiastolite	Promotes balance, harmony and stability. Connects our root chakra to your spiritual center.
Dravite	Brings up negative family patterns in order to deal with them on a spiritual level. Encourages stability and aligning the aura.
Hematite	Helps us to grounding and center while bringing peace and calm.
Jet	Assists with fear issues to bring a sense of serenity and relaxation.
Smoky Quartz	Calms the root chakra to enable grounding and security.

Second Chakra

Bloodstone	Grounds negative energy while removing energy blocks. Cleanses our lower chakras and realigns scattered energy.
Bronzite	Provides essential grounding and protection in situations where we feel powerless. Helps us regain our composure under stressful conditions.
Carnelian	Helps us to stay on center for clear thinking and action. Reinforces our need to stay focused so as not to dwell on things outside of our control.
Moonstone	Promotes a flow of serenity while balancing our emotions. Realigns male/female imbalances.

Red Jasper	Assists us to resolve difficult situations while at the same time helping us to stay grounded and centered. Calms the aura.

Third Chakra

Amber	Draws out feelings of helplessness and unworthiness. Supports a renewed sense of personal worth.
Citrine	Helps to alleviate fear and gives us a feeling of self-empowerment. Supports our ability to manifest our dreams.
Star of the Sea	Takes away everyday worries and concerns to help us understand the bigger picture of the situation confronting us.

Fourth Chakra

Chrysoprase	Calms the heart. Good for hypertension and high blood pressure. Helps us to work out anger issues.
Jade	Transmutes negative energy into positive bringing a sense of peace in order to increase the enjoyment of life.
Kunzite	Natural lithium content helps to lessens anxiety and to show us how to truly love ourselves in order to create the life we desire.
Rhodochrosite	Brings the sweetness and love of Spirit down to our heart chakra to promote unconditional love and joy.
Rose Quartz	Sweet energy which helps to bring a sense of calm. "Grandmother Stone" that says, "There, there, everything is going to be okay."

Fifth Chakra

Amazonite	Calms our chakras and eases aggravation and emotional trauma. Helps us to see both sides of an issue.
Blue Lace Agate	Helps alleviate our feelings of anger so that we can think before we speak. Connects our throat chakra to the crown bringing spiritual energy to the throat chakra.
Chrysocolla	Helps alleviate the fear of being heard. Gently reduces negativity, bringing in a sense of forgiveness. Aligns all of our chakras with the Divine.
Sodalite	Helps us rebalance our emotions by encouraging us to look at a situation with logic to avoid being overly emotional. Gently supports improving our self-esteem and self-acceptance.
Turquoise	A stone of protection that connects our throat chakra to Spirit and to our root chakra. Gives us a sense of security and well-being.

Sixth Chakra

Amethyst	Calming and soothing. Helps us to see a different way to settle things. Provides spiritual guidance and supports development of telepathy.
Angelite	Brings a sense of calm in times of transition and change. Clears our chakras so that a higher vibration of spiritual information may smoothly enter our awareness.
Azurite	Aids in negating negative thinking in order to alleviate worry and stress. Brings up blocked memories to break old patterns and belief systems.
Larimar	Brings a tranquility that allows us to 'go with the flow' to resolve issues. Supports clarity and truth.
Topaz	Replaces negativity with love and joy; stimulates feelings of peace.

Seventh Chakra

Apophyllite	Allows for clear vision and thoughts of a better tomorrow. Helps us to alleviate worry, stress, and fear.
Celestite	A stone of joy and connection to the angelic realms. Reminds us to take things lightly and see the good in all situations.
Fluorite	Assimilates thought patterns helping to calm the mind and bring focus. Clears illusion bringing order into our life.
Howlite	Soothes our emotions by teaching us patience. Helps to relax us in stressful situations. Instills a sense of tranquility to our environment.
Selenite	Clears out old negative patterns and gives us a sense of inner peace. Brings mental clarity in order to relieve stress and anxiety.

Overall

Calcites	Clears out old negative patterns and brings calm to the area being healed. Also frees our mind of 'looping' thoughts to bring clarity and change.
Lepidolite	Natural lithium content gives lepidolite the ability to work on anxiety, stress and tension. Aids in disorders of the nervous system and helps us sleep.
Malachite	Draws out negativity and emotional issues. Helps to discharge buried belief systems and resolve old conditioning in order to move forward in a positive manner.

Resources/Books of Note

Brennan, B., & Smith, J. (2011). Hands of Light. Westminster: Random House Publishing Group.

Walker, D. (1988). The crystal healing book. Pacheco, Calif.: Crystal Co.

Zukav, G., Winfrey, O., & Angelou, M. (1989). The seat of the soul. New York: Simon and Schuster.

Wauters, Ambika (2002). The Book of Chakras: Discover the Hidden Forces Within You. London: New Burlington

Judith, A. (1987). Wheels of Life: A User's Guide to the Chakra System (Llewellyn's New Age Series). Woodbury: Llewellyn Worldwide

Mirdad, M. (2008). You're Not Going Crazy . . . You're Just Waking Up!: The Five Stages of the Soul Transformation Process. Bellingham: Gail Press.

Judith, A. (2004). Eastern Body, Western Mind: Psychology and the Chakra System As a Path to the Self. New York: Crown Publishing Group.

Brown, B. (2010). The Gifts of Imperfection: Let Go of Who You Think You're Supposed to Be and Embrace Who You Are. Center City: Hazelden Publishing. Anthony, C. (2002). Love, an inner connection. Stow, Mass.: Anthony Pub. Co.

Myss, C. (2017). Anatomy of the spirit. New York [New York]: Harmony Books.

Hay, L. (1984). You can heal your life. Carlsbad: Hay House, Inc.

Ruiz, M. (2018). The Four Agreements: A Practical Guide to Personal Freedom (A Toltec Wisdom Book). San Rafael: Amber-Allen Publishing.

Brown, B. (2017). Daring Greatly : How the Courage to Be Vulnerable Transforms the Way We Live, Love, Parent, and Lead. New York: Penguin Random House Audio Publishing Group.

Cohen, A. (2012). Enough already. Carlsbad, Calif.: Hay House.

Thesenga, S., & Pierrakos, E. (2001). The Undefended Self: Living the Pathwork. Charlottesville, Va.: Pathwork Press.

Coelho, P., & Clarke, A. (2014). The Alchemist, 25th Anniversary: A Fable About Following Your Dream. New York: HarperCollins.

Tsabary, S. (2010). The Conscious Parent. Vancouver, Canada: Nameste Publishing.

Bettelheim, B. (1995). A good enough parent. London: Thames & Hudson.

Bloom, D., & Seeman, B. (1999). The KISS Guide to Crystals. Milwaukee: Self-Published.

Bloom, D. (2011). The KISS Guide to Stone Layouts. Milwaukee: Self-Published.

About the Author

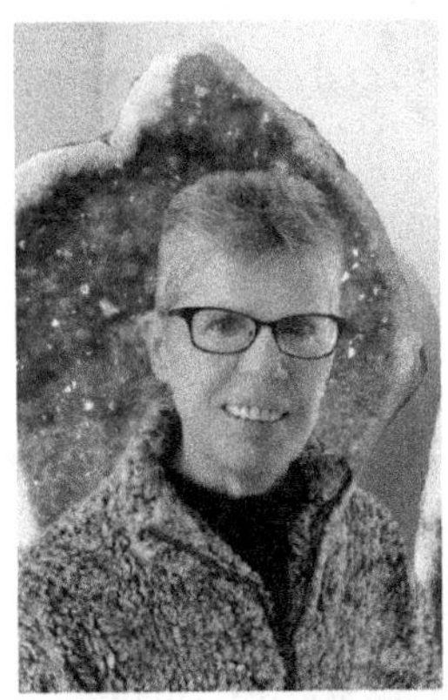

Diane Bloom has a long history of studying with recognized leaders in the crystal community. She began her studies in crystal healing with Katrina Raphaell at the Crystal Academy of Advanced Healing Arts. Soon after, she was accepted to study at Melody's Teacher's School in Denver. Diane is one of only 35 teachers in the world to be initially accredited by Melody to teach her curriculum. As a student of world-renowned Master Crystalogist DaEl Walker, Diane has hosted many learning sessions to provide local students the opportunity to learn crystal healing from him.

Diane is a graduate of The School for Enlightenment and Healing in San Diego headed by Dr. Michael Mamas. She also graduated from Lionheart Institute of Transpersonal Energy Healing in San Antonio and was the co-director of the Milwaukee branch of the school from 2001 to August of 2007.

She established Free Spirit Crystals in the metro Milwaukee area in 1991 and is the co-founder and co-teacher at Free Spirit School of Integrated Energy Healing in Butler,

Wisconsin.

Diane is a Reiki Master-Teacher, a Light Body graduate, Numerologist and has her own healing practice. Diane presents workshops and lectures on healing with stones and energy healing throughout the country. Diane is the author of two books on crystals – The KISS Guide to Crystals and The KISS Guide to Stone Layouts.

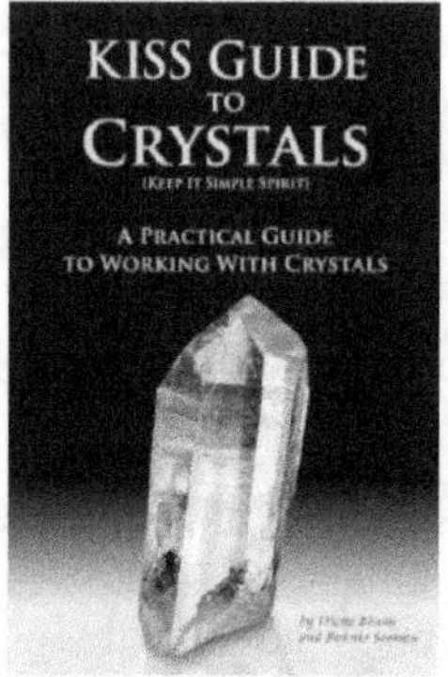

Available for Amazon's Kindle.

Paperback exclusively available from Free Spirit Crystals.

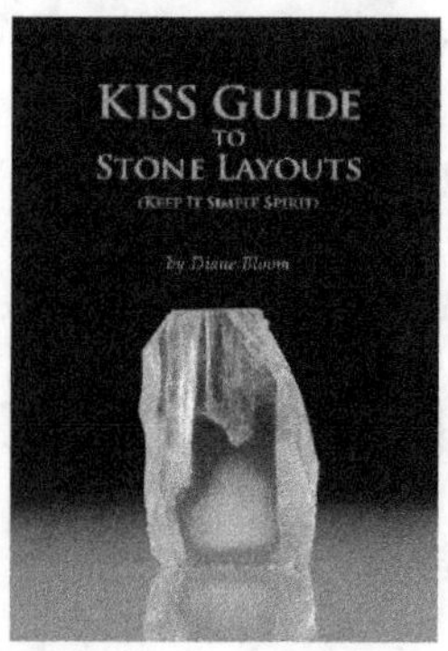

Paperback exclusively available from Free Spirit Crystals.

For more information, contact Diane at freespiritcyrstals@gmail.com or visit her sites online:

Free Spirit Crystals site: http://freespiritcrystals.com

Free Spirit School of Integrated Energy Healing: https://freespiritschool.com/

www.ingramcontent.com/pod-product-compliance
Lightning Source LLC
Chambersburg PA
CBHW081413250726
48654CB00013B/1681